Ask DR. MARIE

Straight Talk and Reassuring Answers
to Your Most Private Questions

MARIE SAVARD, M.D.

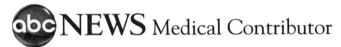 **NEWS** Medical Contributor

with
SONDRA FORSYTH

GUILFORD, CONNECTICUT
An imprint of The Globe Pequot Press

life   GPP Life gives women answers they can trust.

GPP Life is an imprint of The Globe Pequot Press.

ABC News® name and logo are the trademarks of American Broadcasting Companies, Inc., used under express permission by Morris Book Publishing, LLC.

Text design: Sheryl P. Kober
Illustrations: Robert Prince © Morris Book Publishing, LLC

Library of Congress Cataloging-in-Publication Data
Savard, Marie, M.D.
 Ask Dr. Marie : straight talk and reassuring answers to your most private questions / Marie Savard, with Sondra Forsyth.
    p. cm.
 Includes index.
 ISBN 978-0-7627-4944-7
 1. Medicine, Popular. 2. Self-care, Health. 3. Consumer education. I. Forsyth, Sondra. II. Title.
 RC82.S2678 2009
 616—dc22

                                                                         2009010707

Printed in the United States of America

10 9 8 7 6 5 4 3 2 1

*For the men in my life whom I love more than they could know:
my husband, Brad; my three sons, Aaron, Ben, and Zach; and
my father, John*

—Marie Savard, M.D.

*For my son, Christopher; my daughter, Stacey; my son-in-law,
Mark; and my grandson, Shaler*

—Sondra Forsyth

Contents

Contents

Introduction

The Doctor Will See You Now

Let's imagine for a moment that my office door is open. Come on in. We'll close the door so we can have some privacy. You're free to take all the time you need to educate me about yourself, share your concerns and questions, and learn from my knowledge and experience about women's health. Even more important, I want to give you information that will make you marvel at the miracle of your woman's body and inspire you to become your own primary caretaker for every aspect of your health, including prevention, medical records, lifestyle, and decisions about treatment options. After all, who cares more about your health than you do?

Before we begin our ideal office visit, I'm going to take off my white coat and come around from behind my desk to sit in the chair right next to you. I'm a doctor, but I'm also a woman. I want to connect with you as a person who has the same awe-inspiring but sometimes troublesome body parts that you do. I've been in the stirrups for gynecological exams, and I've given those same exams. I've lived the female life cycle of fertility from puberty through pregnancy, childbirth (a firstborn son, followed in short order by twin sons!), breastfeeding, menopause, and life after menopause. Not only that, but I've had my share of problems "down there" as well.

Yet in spite of the fact that I'm a doctor married to a doctor, at times I've been as guilty as the next woman of suffering in silence either because my complaints didn't seem important enough to mention—or because they seemed, well, unmentionable. I've gotten over that as you'll find out when I come forward with my problems in some of the chapters of this book. The point is, though, that even *I* kept these "female troubles" to myself for decades. I have long told each of my patients that whatever questions she has, she is not alone. Yet I had a blind spot when it came to myself. Believe me, opening up has been liberating.

I'll also admit that when I was a young woman, I used to be influenced by the old patriarchal "yes, doctor" model of the physician as an all-knowing authority figure whose wisdom was not to be questioned. That era has long since passed and I've followed my own advice about taking charge of one's health and establishing a doctor-patient relationship based on mutual respect and clear communication. Yet I have become well aware that this is not always easy to put into practice, given the constraints of the health-care system in the United States today. For obvious reasons, office managers and group practice administrators are not pleased with physicians who spend as long with each patient as she truly deserves. (Nor are many physicians themselves, who worry they can't cover their expenses if they see too few patients.)

Consequently, the ideal picture I painted about our long and in-depth consultation in my office would be all but impossible to achieve in reality. That was my impetus for writing this book for you, as an alternative. The idea first came to me back when I was one of four physicians in a group practice with "panels" of thousands of patients. If you had been one of my patients, your visits with me in my office would have been limited to a mere fifteen minutes, which translates to about seven minutes of face time with the doctor, unless you had been scheduled for your annual full physical exam. Even then, we would have had a scant thirty minutes together to cover not only medical issues but everything else you might have liked to confide to me.

If you had been given enough time to relax and open up to me, you might have talked about your sex life, or lack thereof. Or perhaps you would have been honest about the moodiness you had been experiencing at the mercy of hormonal fluctuations, whether as a teenager, a new mother, or a woman entering menopause. If you hadn't felt so rushed, you might even have gotten up the courage to tell me about troubles with your "private parts" that you've been too embarrassed to talk about, such as wetting your pants when you sneeze or cough, straining to have your bowel movements, feeling fat and bloated, or leaking through pads and tampons so that you stain your clothes and sheets. Usually, however, the visit would have been over all too quickly and you would almost certainly have left my office feeling frustrated because only your most urgent or immediate concerns and conditions had been addressed whereas what impacts the day-to-day quality of your life was probably not even considered.

I was frustrated, too, when I was forced to do the medical version of speed dating with my real-life patients. That's why I eventually limited my practice in order to devote most of my working hours to bringing my message of health empowerment to women everywhere.

During my years since then as an author, television and radio commentator, speaker, and consultant, this message has become my mission. At its core it remains the same as it was when I made the decision in medical school to train as an internist rather than as a gynecologist. The year was 1973. Back then there was no formally designated specialty in women's health in the holistic sense of treating the patient instead of just the parts. My first rotation that summer in obstetrics and gynecology made me aware of the gaping need for just such a specialty. I decided that by choosing to become an internist—a "family doctor" who could take care of both men and women—I would get a broad-based medical education that would arm me with the greatest range of knowledge and hands-on experience. Although I wanted to focus on women's health in the long run, I felt strongly that by including men in my practice, I would be better able to understand "all that ails us" as women and to help us help ourselves. That proved to be true as I learned in the trenches day by day during the many years that I had male as well as female patients.

Eventually though, I did begin to concentrate on women's health issues. By 1979, I was a fellow at the University of Colorado having completed an Internal Medicine residency at the University of Pennsylvania. I was looking for a research project. Coincidentally, I had just finished taking a seven-day regimen of antibiotics for a bladder infection called cystitis. I was annoyed at how much trouble it had been for me to find a doctor and get an appointment quickly, and I was also not pleased about the cost of the physical exam, the urinalysis, the urine culture, and week's worth of medications. On top of all that, I was worried that I would end up with a vaginal yeast infection since I knew that the drugs would upset the natural flora of the vagina. Sure enough, I did get yeast vaginitis and then I had to pay for medication to cure that!

Even more important, I had been hesitant about taking the antibiotics because a few years earlier my lab partner and girlfriend during my first year of medical school had died from complications of a severe allergic drug reaction to a sulfa antibiotic that she was taking for cystitis. The drug allergy symptom was a skin rash that was misdiagnosed as a viral infection called pityriasis rosea. She kept on taking the sulfa antibiotic and it eventually killed her. What was so eerie for me was that back then I too had symptoms of cystitis. I was having trouble getting in to see a doctor, so my friend actually gave me her follow-up appointment for the cystitis because she was preoccupied with her newly developed skin condition. No wonder I have spent much of my career teaching women how to manage their own health, how to collect, read, and save their own test results and how important a complete and accurate medical history is. I lost a dear friend years ago in part because she didn't know how important it was for her to be proactive about her health.

Not long after I took the medication for cystitis, I read a research study published in the prominent *New England Journal of Medicine* that reported on how women with symptoms of a urinary tract infection could be accurately diagnosed and successfully, safely, and efficiently treated just on the basis of their response to a three-day course of antibiotics. I learned about a simple method of culturing the urine called the dipslide method, which seemed like a terrific and inexpensive tool that women could use themselves to diagnose their own urinary tract infections (UTIs) at home. They could thus avoid the cost of a doctor's visit and pay only for a short course of antibiotics while minimizing the side effects of medication. Empowering women with information and control was part of my DNA from the beginning, so this study really got me excited! I knew I had found the research area I wanted to devote myself to during my time in Colorado. The results of my study were eventually published in the prestigious *American Journal of Medicine*. The study also launched my career in women's health, patient empowerment, and the use of evidenced-based medicine to inform patients and doctors alike about the best and most cost-effective treatments.

By the mid-1990s I was the director of the Center for Women's Health at the Medical College of Pennsylvania and a regular columnist for *Woman's Day* magazine as a women's health expert. As it happened, I was on the leading edge of this specialty precisely when the recognition in medical circles that women are not just "small men" came at last. I felt somewhat vindicated. I had long been a proponent of treating women with regard to the fact that we metabolize differently from men, that our livers work differently, and that our powerful hormones are sometimes protective and sometimes a challenge to our overall brain and body well-being. Soon I became an advisor to the spanking-new Subcommittee on Clinical Competency in Women's Health of the American Board of Internal Medicine.

Because I'm not a gynecologist but rather an internist with a specialty in women's health, my expertise about the strictly female concerns of the area "below the belt" is informed by my in-depth knowledge of the body as a whole and my awareness of the potent mind/body connection. As you may know, the phrase "below the belt" comes from a boxing rule that prohibits hitting a man's groin. What's interesting is that in the 1970s when women's boxing became a professional sport, the "below the belt rule" was applied to women as well, in order to protect the womb. Male and female boxers alike now wear external protectors so that there's less chance of damage to the organs we need in order to conceive. I like the idea that we should also learn to protect our precious area internally with good health knowledge and habits rather taking a chance on harming it with life choices that "hit below the belt."

There is also a general lack of understanding about what really goes on "down there" and a good measure of mortification about the often smelly, sticky, itchy, leaky symptoms of what we still refer to among ourselves as "female troubles." That's the reason I chose to make our internal female organs and our "plumbing" the main focus of this book. I do make some references to our breasts, but only when issues concerning them are intrinsically tied to the functions and problems of our mysterious inner gynecological landscape.

Having said all of that, I want to add that I started my career in medicine as a nurse. During my years on the wards and in an intensive care unit as a critical-care nurse, I had the opportunity to develop personal connections with patients. I cared about them and I wanted to be an advocate for them. That was the beginning of my lifelong passion for patient power.

A turning point in my life came in an ICU late one night when a sweet, frail woman in her eighties with a brain tumor began the violent, rhythmic convulsions typical of a grand mal seizure. I knew she needed intravenous Valium, and fast. However, as a nurse I was not legally allowed to administer the medication without a doctor's verbal order. I called for the intern on duty and then waited what seemed like an eternity while the woman continued to twitch and shake uncontrollably. Finally a very young doctor, groggy from the sleep deprivation typical of all residents, arrived and insisted on doing a brief examination rather than take my word for what was happening. I felt utterly powerless and demeaned. In that moment, I knew without a doubt that I was going to find a way to go back to school and become a full-fledged physician. Like the vast majority of women of my generation and my mother's generation before me, I had seen teaching and nursing as my only two career options. My mother herself was a nurse and I followed her example. Yet my epiphany that night in the ICU in 1970, bolstered by the rebirth of American feminism that was under way, spurred me to enter the almost-all-male preserve of M.D.s. Looking back, I see that I knew even then that my mission would be to empower women as the guardians and nurturers of their own health.

To that end, women must understand their bodies and be tuned in to their personal health. I urge you to honor your intuition and emotions, including not giving anyone else's opinion or needs higher billing than your own, be it a partner pressuring you for sex or a doctor disregarding your questions and concerns. The "Golden Rule" asks us to "Do unto others as you would do unto yourself." I would argue that for women, we need to flip that around so that it says, "Do unto yourself as you would do unto others."

What I mean is that you need to take care of yourself with at least as much devotion as you take care of everybody else. We tend to put ourselves last on our list of priorities but that's not good for those we love any more than it's good for us.

My "Golden Rule of Women's Health" applies to all of us at all ages and stages of our lives. Are you a teen who's only recently started getting your period? Are you a woman in your childbearing years? Are you a woman approaching or going through menopause? Are you a woman enjoying the decades of life after menopause that were denied to so many of our grandmothers and even our mothers before medical advances dramatically upped our life expectancy? Whatever the case, the following pages offer clear, comprehensive, and compassionate answers to your questions about sex, libido, hormones, and everything else that goes on "down there." You'll hear the voices of real women dishing about the intimate and sometimes funny details of everything from birth control to bladder problems to menopause. I'll give you lists of symptoms so you'll know whether to get help for those aches and itches and discharges and bumps. You'll also find:

- straight talk about what I call Smart Sex
- lists of diagnostic tests including those you can do yourself
- solid medical advice about treatment options ranging from over-the-counter and home remedies to surgery
- translations of medical jargon into language you can understand
- examples of actual medical test results
- sketches to help you understand once and for all what's going on "down there"
- advice about how to get the most out of the doctor/patient relationship
- plenty of encouragement to help you find a fresh and positive perspective about the inevitable transformations you'll encounter as you enter each new chapter of your life

In many ways, this book is even better than that hypothetical office visit I asked you to imagine. You can come back to these pages again and again whenever a symptom or a life change or a treatment decision prompts you to look for information and reassurance. You can also share the information across the generations in your family and among your friends. Women have instinctively been one another's "health buddies," confidantes, soothers, and healers since the dawn of human history. Now more than ever, as we are bombarded by information technology and hurried through our health-care consultations and procedures, we need to help each other by sharing our stories truthfully and becoming fully informed about our health as women.

Let's celebrate our bodies for the wonders of nature that they are. For one thing, they give us a statistical edge over men in the longevity department. They also give us the chance to choose to savor the pleasures of sex, to bring the next generation of babies into the world, and to nourish those babies with mother's milk. However, even if you are a woman who isn't willing or able to fulfill any of those biological functions—and I respect your life circumstances and choices 100 percent—you need to appreciate the marvel of your female body and learn how to keep it healthy. For example, the elderly nuns I treat as the primary care physician for the Cabrini Retirement and Nursing Home in Philadelphia need every bit as much care of their female organs and their "plumbing" as do women who have been sexually active and given birth.

Cabrini was the crucible of my crusade for patient power, in particular the need to collect your own medical records. When I first arrived there in 1981, the missionary sisters were overmedicated and their records were literally scattered all over the world, with most of the paperwork still in their mission countries. As I gradually gathered together what I needed to make accurate diagnoses and treat these women properly, I devised a method of record keeping that turned out to be the genesis of the Savard System I first made available in 2000 and which I continue to refine to this day. With the nuns' records well organized, I was able to help them benefit from the most alert, vigorous, and pain-free lives possible.

That's what I want for all of us. When we're healthy women in control of our wellness, we are far better able to sharpen our minds, pursue gainful employment, and just plain have a terrific time being alive with our partners, our children, our extended families, our colleagues, and our dear friends. That's why I want you to get past any reservations you may have about tuning in to your total self. I want you to do all you can to achieve optimum health as much as is possible for you. You owe that to yourself and to those who love you.

Let's start with a guided tour of the hidden treasures in your body that define your womanhood. . . .

PART I

What's Going On Down There?

1
Welcome to Yourself

A Guided Tour of Your Inner Terrain

IN THIS CHAPTER

- Your Female Reproductive Organs
- Inner Plumbing Down There: Your Urinary Tract
- Inner Plumbing Down There: Your Bowels

Warning: Contains adult language. No, I don't mean four-letter words and their ilk. I mean the grown-up words for female body parts that I learned in medical school. I'm not going to use coy euphemisms such as "va-jay-jay" for vagina. I'm a doctor and you're an adult. Well, okay, maybe you're a teenager. But if you're old enough to menstruate, you're physically a woman and you don't have to resort to baby talk any more than the rest of us do. Whatever your age, I'm here to share with you a tour of the miraculous organs that make us women. We don't need silly, made-up words that diminish the majesty of those organs.

Wow! That was pretty stern coming from me! You know from reading the introduction or watching me on *Good Morning America* that I'm the polar opposite of the high-and-mighty physician who talks down to patients and doesn't invite questions or discussions. I'm more like your best friend who also happens to be a doctor. But that's exactly why I'm so determined to encourage you to embrace the real vocabulary for our womanly anatomy. I want you to be completely comfortable with yourself and to be able to talk with your own doctor—and for that matter with your mother, your daughters, your friends, and your partners—without any hint of embarrassment.

That said, I actually don't mind if you refer to the whole female genital area as "down there" because that's what we've been saying for generations and it's good shorthand with no cutesy or negative connotations. I don't even mind if you say "private parts" because they are in fact private in the sense of being off-limits to anyone else unless you agree to be seen and touched there. There are perfectly good terms for the organs and functions of what's "down there," and using those terms imbues us with a feeling of respect and even wonder about our bodies rather than shame and ignorance. Let's leave words such as va-jay-jay and wee-wee to the nursery school set—although plenty of parents these days even teach their little ones to use the real terms right from the start.

Of course, baby-talk words for female private parts aren't the only euphemisms around. There's a whole arsenal of slang terms used almost exclusively by men. Those words are downright derogatory at worst and cloyingly paternalistic at best. On the other hand, slang terms for penis, again used largely by men, suggest either power or a kind of hail-fellow-well-met camaraderie. Plenty of men even name their penises as though they were alter egos.

Why are we so much less likely than men to think of our genitalia as a positive part of our identity? Perhaps the reason is that even our outer genitalia are tucked in to the point that we need to wield a mirror to get a glimpse of them. But "private" should not equal mysterious, and it certainly should not equal embarrassing. Also, Freud's theory of "penis envy" notwithstanding, I've never known any woman who feels that the lack of readily visible reproductive body parts makes her jealous of what men have! Women, after all, possess the parts with the potential not just to get the procreational process going but to bring it to fruition if they choose and are able to do that. Most of us do feel that the uterus defines us as women, for better or for worse. As one of my patients said, "When I had a miscarriage, I took it personally. When I finally got pregnant again but then had to have a scheduled C-section because I was way past my due date, I took it personally. I mean, if I had trouble with my gall bladder, I would just think of it as an organ that didn't work right. When something goes wrong with my uterus, I feel like a failure."

She's not alone, and of course the flip side is that women feel pride when everything from conception to labor and delivery goes well. But my goal is to have us achieve, regardless of our individual experiences with our bodies, a profound appreciation for what we have inside—not only our reproductive organs but also the urinary tract and gastrointestinal tract. Collectively, they amount to a breathtakingly beautiful and intricate biological ballet. I think that's cause for celebration. Once you've taken the following tour, I'm confident you'll agree.

YOUR FEMALE REPRODUCTIVE ORGANS

Anatomy textbooks typically start with the innermost female organs—the ovaries—and go on from there organ by organ until they finally describe the external parts. That seems backwards to me. I'm going to start at the entrance and take you from there on a journey to your terra incognita.

OPEN SESAME: THE VULVA

When most people say "vagina"—if they say it at all rather than using a euphemism such as "va-jay-jay"—they actually mean the vulva. The vulva is not an organ but a region. It includes the external organs of the female reproductive system. Grab a hand-held mirror, shut yourself in the bathroom, and take off your panties. Sit on the toilet and spread your legs or simply stand in a straddle position. Position the mirror between your legs and have a look. Here's what you'll see:

Mons Pubis

This term, translated from the Latin, means "pubic mountain." It's the little fleshy bulge over your pubic bone—a convenient built-in shock absorber designed to cushion you during your partner's thrusts when you're having sex. Another term for the mons pubis is "mons veneris," meaning "Venus's mountain." Hey, it's good to be a goddess! Finally, it's also called the "pubic eminence." "Eminence" is a medical term for any protrusion. But why not think instead about "eminence" with the meaning "a person of high rank and superiority"? That describes you perfectly, right? I'm only half kidding. No less an authority than the Mayo Clinic devotes a page on their Web site to encouraging "positive self-talk" as a route to increased self-esteem.

Oh, and while I'm at it I need to mention that whatever you choose to call this mound of flesh, it gets covered with hair when you hit puberty. Or not. We're all different and you may grow lots of hair that even extends back toward your anus, or your pubic hair may be sparse. Most women find that pubic hair thins and gets a little coarser after

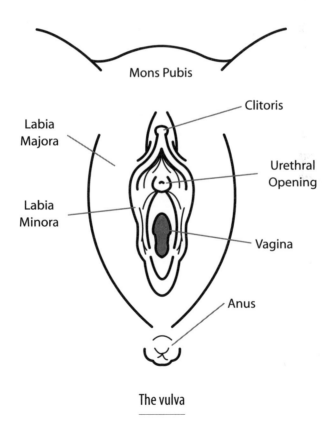

The vulva

menopause. It also turns gray with age. (My waxer tells me that some of her clients dye their pubic hair. Don't do that! You shouldn't risk getting dye on your sensitive genital tissues and perhaps causing inflammation or infection.)

Some women go for a "bikini waxing" (I'm one of them) and still others opt for a so-called "Brazilian" that removes all the hair in the pubic region except sometimes for a central strip. Yes, a Brazilian hurts. Yes, it's expensive. The procedure was introduced in New York in 1987 by seven Brazilian sisters and became all the rage in the 1990s. The results last about six weeks. If your bathing suit is revealing enough to show the hair in your nether region, you might consider getting a Brazilian. However, you should know that your pubic hair helps "soften the blow," so to speak, during sex. Also, we each have a personal scent that can turn men on. Your pubic hair captures your unique fragrance.

Labia Majora

The term is Latin for "larger lips" and it refers to the pair of darkish pink or brownish skin folds that you can see in your handheld mirror right below your mons pubis. The opening between the lips is the entrance to your vagina. This entrance is sometimes called the Cleft of Venus— another nod to the goddess of love! However, it is also called the "pudendal fissure." Believe it or not, the Latin meaning of "pudendal" is "ashamed." Some male doctor eons ago must have picked that name! In the nineteenth century, pelvic exams were rarely done because doctor and patient alike were embarrassed by the procedure. Aren't you glad that we no longer need to be embarrassed by what's "down there"?

Labia Minora

On the other hand, some women are now embarrassed in a different way. They think their vulvae aren't pretty enough, especially if the labia minora ("smaller lips") protrude through the labia majora. In what has been dubbed the "designer vagina" craze, women are flocking to plastic

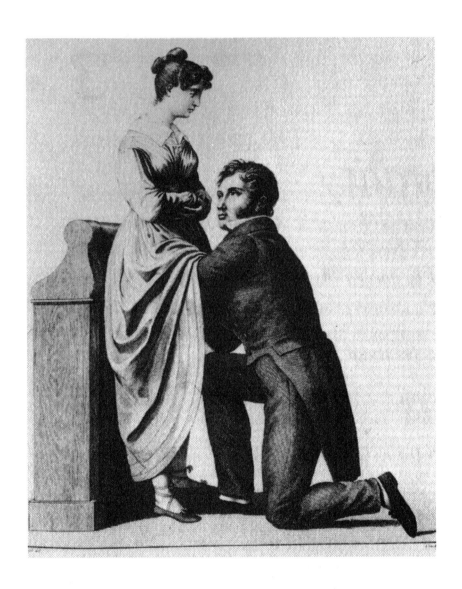

A nineteenth-century male doctor performing a pelvic examination surgeons for a surgical technique called labiaplasty. A 2005 report in the prestigious *British Medical Journal* sounded an alarm that the procedure is untested and may result in problems with sexual arousal. My take on this trend? Do not have this potentially risky elective cosmetic surgery. (If there's a new man in your life who is turned off by how you look down there, he's not the one for you. Basing a relationship on the appearance of your vulva hardly bodes well for a loving and lasting union!)

Clitoris

Just inside the labia minora and near the top of them, you'll see your clitoris and its hood. The clitoris is a miniature version of a man's penis. In this case, though, size really doesn't matter. Your little bulb of erectile tissue is extremely sensitive and it's capable of giving you powerful orgasms (see chapter 2, page 24.) Linguists are still debating the origin of the word "clitoris," but I'm in the camp with those who believe it comes from the Greek verb "kleitoriazein," meaning "to tickle and to be inclined toward pleasure."

Vestibule of the Vagina

Right behind your clitoris is what you can think of as the entrance hall or foyer to the openings of your vagina and your urethra.

Bartholin's Glands

Named for the seventeenth-century anatomist Caspar Bartholin the Younger, who first described the glands, they generate droplets of lubricating mucus when you are sexually aroused. However, most of the lubrication you experience during sex comes not from mucus but from body fluids that are forced into your vagina as a result of the engorgement of blood vessels. The Bartholin's glands are on either side of the entrance to the vagina.

Hymen

You may or may not have been born with one of the many versions of this translucent mucous membrane that can stretch across the entrance to the vagina. The origin of the term is the name of the Greek god of marriage, Hymenaios. Generations of women all over the world have long believed that on the wedding night, the groom can tell whether the bride has remained a virgin because a spot of blood on the sheets will prove that her hymen has ruptured with her first incidence of intercourse. Some plastic surgeons offer a "hymenoplasty" to repair a torn hymen, especially for women whose cultures and religions are so adamant about an intact hymen as evidence of a woman's respectability that they perform "honor killings." A bride who did not stain the sheets is sacrificed to restore honor to her family. However, the truth is that some women have no hymen and others have one that stretches but never breaks. Stretching without bleeding can happen during first intercourse or it can happen during physical activity such as gymnastics or riding a bike, or when a tampon is inserted. (Inserting a tampon will not break your hymen.) In other words, you're a certifiable virgin if your "cherry pops" the first time you have sex but you may not see any blood even if you are a virgin.

INWARD TO THE CHAMBER OF PROCREATION AND WOMANLY WELL-BEING

You can put your mirror down now. We've completed our tour of the external organs. The rest are deeper inside you.

Vagina

The vagina is a muscular tube about four inches long that leads to the uterus. This tube is lined with mucous membranes similar to those in your mouth except that the vagina isn't smooth. It's a series of folds designed to allow the tube to expand or contract. That's why your vagina can accept your partner's penis during sex and adjust for a snug fit no

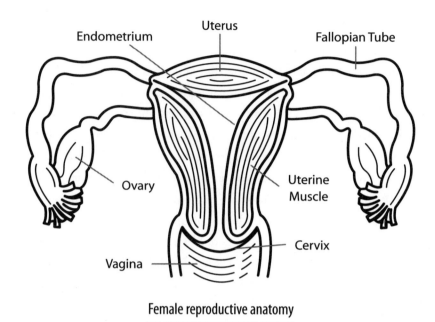

Female reproductive anatomy

matter what the size of his penis may be. Your vagina can also close around any size tampon. But that's not all! This amazing passageway can balloon so that it's big enough to be the "birth canal" for the delivery of a full-term baby. Let's hear a round of applause for the vagina, an organ of many talents!

After experiencing an expanding event, the vagina contracts or tightens again so that its opening is a mere slit. No matter how many times you have sex or use a tampon or give birth, your vagina will not become "loose." The muscles of your pelvic sling may slacken, but the vagina itself doesn't change enough to make any difference in your sexual pleasure or your partner's. Plastic surgeons offer "vaginal rejuvenation" or tightening, but you're better off doing Kegel exercises for the muscles of your pelvic floor and avoiding the risks of going under the knife for a dubious procedure that may compromise the functions of your vagina. (See chapter 9, page 290, for an explanation of how to do Kegel exercises.)

Cervix

The word literally means "neck" in Latin. Your cervix is the entrance to your uterus. The "donut hole," a term I coined to describe the opening of the cervix, has two kinds of cells. Those near the opening are flat "squamous" cells. The ones next to the uterus are tall "columnar" cells. In between, there is a "transformation zone" where columnar cells are continually transformed into squamous cells. This zone, unfortunately, is a hospitable environment for viruses, primarily human papillomavirus (HPV), which can lead to abnormal cell changes and possibly cervical cancer (see chapter 2, page 44). In girls and young women, the transformation zone is on the outside of the opening of the donut hole. In older women it's farther inside. That's why younger women are more prone to infections, including HPV.

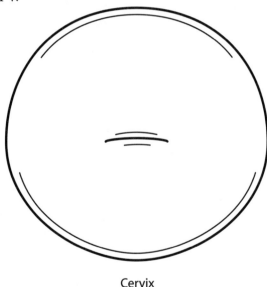

Cervix

The "donut hole" of the cervix

Uterus

Also called the womb, from the Latin for "belly," your uterus is a hollow, somewhat triangular cavity with muscular walls. The lining of

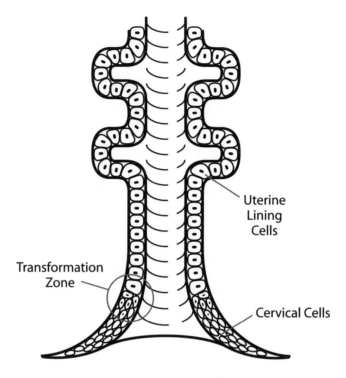

The transformation zone of the cervix

the uterus is a membrane called the endometrium. During your menstrual cycle the endometrium thickens with blood vessels. These are eventually shed with menstruation if you don't get pregnant. During a pregnancy the endometrium thickens even more while the fetus develops.

Fallopian Tubes
Also called the "oviducts," these tubes lead to your ovaries. The fallopian tubes are named after the sixteenth-century Italian physician and anatomist Gabriele Falloppio. There is one tube on either side of the triangle of the uterus. Inside the tubes there are little hairlike organs called cilia that push eggs down toward the uterine cavity, where they

can be fertilized. (See chapter 7, page 222 for information about potential problems with the fallopian tubes.)

Ovaries

We've now arrived at your innermost female organs, the ovaries. These two little nodes, one on either side of your uterus, are in the neighborhood of your fallopian tubes but not attached to them. Ovaries weigh in at less than one-tenth of an ounce each, but they have two important functions. They are storehouses for ova, or eggs, and they are also powerhouses of hormones that are essential for a woman's emotional and physical well-being. These hormones are especially potent during the fertile years but they are still produced in vital quantities by the

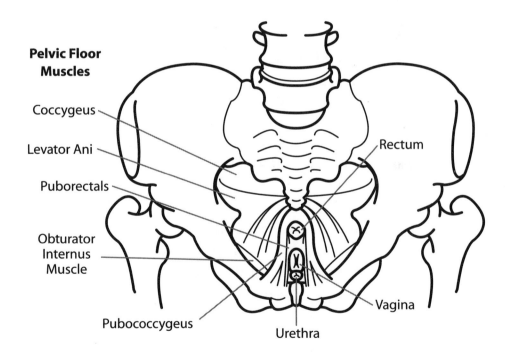

The "pelvic sling"—female pelvis and pelvic floor anatomy

ovaries after menopause. (See "Hysterectomies" in chapter 7, page 231, for information about why a radical hysterectomy, which removes the ovaries, may not be a wise treatment option.)

A female fetus at twenty weeks already has a whopping 7.5 million ova maturing in her ovaries. Nobody knows why we need that many potential eggs, but it's safe to say that our odds for survival of the species are pretty good given such an ample supply. After a female baby is born, the number of ova plummets to about two million, and by puberty a girl typically has around 300,000 eggs. (See chapter 5, page 157 and chapter 6, page 176 for more about the natural decrease in the number of ova during the fertile years and into menopause.)

That concludes our journey to the center of your female organs. Impressed? I am. What a miracle of nature we are! Now I'll give you the information you need in order to understand your urinary tract and your bowels. That way you'll be well versed in the relevant terminology when we get to the chapters about problems in those areas.

INTERNAL PLUMBING DOWN THERE: YOUR URINARY TRACT

URETHRA

This is the tube that has an opening that allows you to urinate. It's one of your "three holes"—the urethra, the vagina, and the anus—all of which are close enough together that bacteria and infections can migrate pretty easily from one to the other. (See chapters 7, 8, and 9 for more on this topic.)

BLADDER

This is your personal storage bag for urine.

URETERS

These tubes lead up from your bladder to your kidneys.

KIDNEYS

These admirably complex and crucial organs work to excrete waste products called urea and uric acid from your body. They also help regulate your metabolism and blood pressure, among other functions. (See chapter 9 for information about tests and treatment options for kidney problems.)

INTERNAL PLUMBING DOWN THERE: YOUR BOWELS

ANUS

This is the opening at the end of your digestive tract through which you have your bowel movements. There is a transformation zone between the internal and external tissues where high-risk strains of HPV such as HPV 16 can remain dormant for years and eventually cause cancer.

BOWELS

They are also called the intestines. The small bowel continues the process of digestion after food leaves the stomach, and the large bowel, or colon, finishes the job.

RECTUM

This is the end of your large intestine where your solid waste, or stool, is stored before you are ready to have a bowel movement. (See chapter 8 for information on bowel problems and treatment options.)

Okay, class dismissed! We made it through the all-important but sometimes eye-glazing anatomy lecture. Now we get to have a little fun. Coming right up, the sex chapter!

2

Sex Smarts

The Thinking Woman's Guide to Having Fun in Bed

IN THIS CHAPTER

- The Science of Desire

- But What about Pleasure?

- The Masters and Johnson Era

- Your Orgasms Demystified

- How Sex Keeps You Healthy and Happy

- The Case for Do-It-Yourself Sex

- Libido Boosters from Rhinoceros Horns to Hormones

- Libido Busters

- Sexually Transmitted Infections (STIs)

- Bacterial Infections

Sex, when all is as it should be, can be one of life's greatest sources of physical and emotional well-being. Think of the sweet urgency of a first kiss. The pulsing pleasure of a mutual orgasm. The sense of serenity when you're cradled in one another's arms in the afterglow. The satisfaction of knowing it was good for your partner, too. Yet unless you have what I call Sex Smarts, enjoying moments such as those may be frustratingly elusive. Worse yet, you may be putting your health at risk.

But I know what you're thinking: What can she possibly tell me about sex that I haven't already heard? After all, ours is a sex-saturated society. Mainstream magazines displayed at child's-eye level at the supermarket checkout counter tempt readers with promises that border on the pornographic ("The Hottest Sex Position Yet! You'll Both *Explode!*," "Down and Dirty Tricks That Will Drive Him Wild"). Billboards, television commercials, and ads for print and Web publications use sex to sell. Movies rated PG-13 leave it up to the parents of tweens and teens whether or not to heed warnings such as "sexual content," "nudity," and "crude sexual language." Not only that, but in the almost five decades since the Pill gave women reproductive freedom and spawned the Sexual Revolution, taboos have fallen one after another. These days, couples who don't live together before marriage are the exception rather than the rule. The vast majority of girls have their "sexual debut" while still in their teens. Oral and anal sex are so common that many girls consider themselves "technical virgins" if they've done "everything but." Finally, sex education starting at least in middle school if not earlier—and I've taught those courses—surely arms the members of each new generation with all they need to know about the subject. Right?

Wrong. The results of sex education in the schools are dubious at best. A study done by the Centers for Disease Control and Prevention in 2008 reported that fully one-quarter of teenage girls in the "hookup generation" have contracted sexually transmitted infections ranging from annoying genital warts to the potentially fatal forms of the human papillomavirus that can cause cervical cancer as well as oral and anal cancer. Plus, teenage pregnancy rates continue to rise, fueled perhaps by celebrity magazines that feature unwed teen idols cradling adorable newborns and gushing about how cool it is to be a mommy.

As for adults, during my twenty-five years of medical practice, I've been privy to the intimate problems and questions that women of all ages still have about sex. The glossies and the tabloids don't teach women what they really need to know. Madison Avenue with its Photoshopped images and clever marketing slogans doesn't give women realistic information or advice. Movies most often present romanticized versions of sexual encounters and may even glorify such issues as multiple sex partners, teenage pregnancy, and unprotected sex. What's more, people who grew up after the sexual mores shifted in this country were navigating uncharted physical and emotional waters. I know from those who have been my patients that many of them foundered when it came to the issues involved in sexuality.

So, yes, I believe there is a great deal that I have to tell you about sex that you probably haven't heard before—at least not in depth and not in a way that can put you at ease with subjects that continue to make most women uncomfortable. As with every aspect of your health, I want you to be knowledgeable and in control. Honestly though, there was a time when I never thought I'd say that. The year that the FDA approved the Pill for use as a contraceptive—1960—I was a good little eleven-year-old Catholic schoolgirl. Along with my classmates—and for that matter most of my generation, whether Catholic or not—I was taught that sex was for procreation only and that you should "save yourself" for marriage. The "Make Love, Not War" years of the 1960s gave way to the new feminism of the early 1970s by the time I reached adulthood. I was never really caught up in the seismic shifts of the era of "free love" and flower children. When I enrolled in medical school at the University of Pennsylvania in 1972 at the age of 23, the idea that I might end up studying human sexuality never entered my head.

I was in for a surprise. Harold Lief, M.D., a pioneer in the field of sex education and therapy, was one of my professors. He was a leading advocate of including sexual education in the training of physicians. His 1976 textbook, *Sex Education in Medicine*, was groundbreaking at the time and went on to become a classic. Penn's program would eventually train scores of therapists in this burgeoning field. Yet as a blushing first-year medical student, one of only a handful of women in classrooms full of men, I was shocked and embarrassed when we watched Dr. Lief's documentary film with graphic video clips of couples going through the steps of normal sexual relationships and of couples who were seeking therapy because they had problems. On camera a medical student admits, "I would never ask an old person about sex." "What's old?" Lief wants to know. "Anyone

42 or over," the student replies. I vividly remember thinking at the time that I couldn't imagine asking *anyone*, regardless of age, about sex! In actual practice though, this course stood me in good stead. Even as a young doctor, I recognized how important knowing about a patient's sex life could be in treating the whole person.

Sex is the hallmark of a relationship. It assures the future of our species and is just plain important for our physical, mental, and emotional health. Yet perhaps none of us thinks we have it just right. We may wish we had better sex lives and a stronger interest in sex. We may wish that we enjoyed it more, that we had more and better orgasms (or any orgasms at all), that we didn't make excuses, or that we didn't go to bed before our partners do. (*Monday Night Football* often ends when I'm already fast asleep because I have to get up early for my commute to work.) Does that sound all too familiar? You're not alone. I'm here to reassure you and help you have the most fulfilling sex life you can with the least possible harm. Let's start with learning about the biology that makes us tick as sexual beings.

THE SCIENCE OF DESIRE

On the most rudimentary level, sex is for making babies. Like every other class of creatures on the planet, we are hardwired to mate with members of the opposite gender who seem to hold the promise of producing healthy offspring that will ensure our part in the survival of the species. And unlike some other species, we also require that our partners in propagation stick around long enough to nurture and support our progeny throughout what has become a dramatically extended adolescence.

Researchers have done countless studies on this topic with conclusions that pretty much detail the obvious. To wit, men in general are attracted to full-breasted women in their prime who have generous hips and are therefore apparently good candidates for birthing and breastfeeding. (The truth, though, is that while we do need fairly wide hips, we don't necessarily need an ample bosom. I am all but flat, yet I breastfed twins successfully!) Women are drawn to men who look and act mature enough to be able to pay the orthodontia bills and the college tuition. Not that a guy who ogles an amply endowed prospect thinks to himself, "Wow, she'll probably have an easy labor and nurse the kid until he's three!" And a woman who gets all flirty with a guy who's buff but has a touch of gray at the temples is not consciously lighting up whatever part of her brain it is that sends the signal "Good provider! Good provider!" When we're drawn to someone at the beginning of a potential courtship, we're not consciously aware that the powerful hormones dopamine, serotonin, and adrenaline are creating an inner cocktail that causes us to gravitate toward a collaborator in procreation who's the most likely to succeed. Still, the scientific explanation for what attracts us to a good catch during the reproductive years hardly comes as a shock.

Research has also brought to our attention another no-surprise-here finding: Preening and displays of come-hither behavior in the animal kingdom are not unlike our own. Peacocks fan their tails, cockatiels do a mating dance, toadfish sing a love song, and female butterflies send out titillating blue flashes of light from their wings. As for homo sapiens, the men among us strut and swagger and pay arguably as much attention to getting six-pack abs and cultivating just the right amount sex-appeal beard stubble as we do to stalking the cosmetic aisles, coping with cellulite, and engaging in such apparently innate and universal attention-getters as batting our eyelashes, giggling, and licking our lips.

BUT WHAT ABOUT PLEASURE?

You know as well as I do that human beings are vastly more complex than, say, a cat in heat or the famously monogamous prairie vole. While the research I referred to highlights the stereotypes of men and women in the courtship phase, our sex lives as females are not at all limited to that most basic goal of going forth and multiplying. We also seek—and in fact *need*—the pleasure that sex can bring us at virtually any age, whether we are aiming for pregnancy, trying to avoid it, are no longer fertile, or are engaging in sex with another woman. The female orgasm, after all, is purely for pleasure. Men do enjoy their orgasms, but the penis ejaculates for a purpose. The clitoris, on the other hand, our dainty but remarkably similar erectile counterpart, is all about feel-good swelling and pulsing that is entirely unrelated to the biological imperative for copulation. Of course, the pleasure we get from orgasms may keep us coming back for more, and that would improve the odds of reproducing during the childbearing years. However, we can get pregnant without having an orgasm, meaning the clitoris is only peripherally necessary for procreation. And recent studies have debunked the myth that older women eschew sex. Many women well into their seventies are still enjoying great sex, thank you very much. Considering all of that, if whatever higher power you may believe in didn't want you to have fun with your sensuous little clitoris, she wouldn't have given it to you!

Did I really just say that? I have indeed come a long way from the girl I was when I was growing up in the 1950s. I clearly recall my mom telling me about sex and having babies. "You see," she said, "God plants a little seed. . . ." I thought he somehow planted the seeds in our belly buttons and then things simply took off from there. It was how that seed got planted that my mother would have been way too embarrassed to describe, and she certainly wouldn't have admitted that there was any pleasure involved—least of all pleasure for its own sake! (A precocious ten-year-old at Girl Scout camp gave me at least a little more information when she whispered in my ear that the man actually puts "that thing" inside you to plant the seed.)

KINSEY'S *SEXUAL BEHAVIOR IN THE HUMAN FEMALE*

My limited introduction to sexuality notwithstanding, the University of Indiana's Alfred C. Kinsey had published his pioneering 1953 book, *Sexual Behavior in the Human Female*, six years before my summer at Girl

Scout camp. Kinsey's research (which had also led to the publication in 1948 of his *Sexual Behavior in the Human Male*) resulted in a first-ever report about such hitherto taboo subjects as female masturbation, female premarital sex, female orgasms, and lesbian liaisons.

According to an article published by the university commemorating the 50th anniversary of the 1953 book, "As expected, public reaction ranged from admiration and gratitude to horror and disgust." But there was no turning back. Kinsey, however flawed and primitive his data collection methods may have been, had succeeded in putting front and center his firm belief that there is no basis for dualism between normal and abnormal sexuality and that, in the words of Dr. Judith A. Allen, a professor in Indiana University's Gender Studies Program, "if a behavior or characteristic could appear in a species, then it was a natural part of that species."

In my view, this is all the more astonishing given the fact that Kinsey observed more than 1,000 couples having sex *in their homes in Indiana in the late 1940s!* Why couples agreed to participate in that place and at that time remains something of a mystery. My best guess is that the war was over, the baby boom generation was being born, and people were somehow ready to open up about the most private of activities in the most private of locations—their own bedrooms. The cloud of secrecy that surrounded Kinsey's work left him open to attacks by critics, and shortly before his death in 1956, he sealed his files. Not until the 50th anniversary of his 1948 book did the University of Indiana publish a collection called "The Kinsey Data" with the aim of vindicating his research and methodology. Some of his critics were mollified. Others were not. But none of them could change the fact that he had opened the Pandora's box that had been kept closed for so long.

KINSEY VS. FREUD

Kinsey considered himself to be an empirical researcher and he railed against Sigmund Freud's less scientifically based theories that were in vogue at the time. Leaving aside Freud's sweeping definition of sexual desire as the top motivator—for better or for worse—of human life, the one assertion that really irked Kinsey was Freud's Victorian-era belief that although the clitoris was capable of being a source of pleasure for little girls, the vagina became preeminent once a woman began to have sexual relations with a man. Kinsey's crusade to debunk the myth of the vaginal orgasm as the only desirable (and, most people infer, respectable) one for a married woman was carried on after Kinsey's death by the team of sex researchers who dominated the field from the late 1950s through the 1990s.

THE MASTERS AND JOHNSON ERA

Gynecologist William Masters, M.D. picked up where Kinsey left off. He started a program on human sexuality at Washington University in St. Louis in 1957. Soon after that he hired psychologist Virginia Johnson as a researcher. They became known to all as Masters and Johnson. (Masters eventually divorced his first wife to marry Johnson in 1969.) They established an independent, not-for-profit research institution in St. Louis in 1964 that came to be called the Masters and Johnson Institute. The team remained professional and personal partners until their divorce in 1993. She retired before the divorce and he retired in 1994. Their publications included *Human Sexual Response* (1966), *Human Sexual Inadequacy* (1970), *Homosexuality in Perspective* (1979), and *Heterosexual Behavior in the Age of AIDS* (1988).

By focusing on the biology of sex, Masters and Johnson confirmed that the vaginal orgasm is not the most important criterion for an adult female's satisfying sex life. All of their patients got a physical exam on their first day at the clinic. They then engaged in sexual intercourse or masturbation so that their sexual response could be studied. For the female patients, Masters used a tiny camera to take pictures inside the vagina in order to document the response.

Some of their patients were perimenopausal or postmenopausal women complaining of decreased libido. These patients were typically prescribed a combination of estrogen and testosterone.

The research of Masters and Johnson, and of Kinsey who preceded them, dovetailed perfectly with the Sexual Revolution of the same era. Thanks to them, we have scientific information about what the "Big O" really is. For the record, these researchers made no mention of the debatable "G-spot," which is named after German gynecologist Ernst Gräfenberg, or the questionable "female ejaculation" it purportedly can produce. As a physician myself with a thorough knowledge of anatomy, I think there's plenty of pleasure to be had with the organs we actually possess.

Here then, is what the work of Masters and Johnson taught us:

WHAT IS AN ORGASM ANYWAY?

Masters and Johnson identified four phases of the female sexual response. They also noted that while men experience a "refractory period" after an orgasm when they can't ejaculate again, women have no refractory period and can have multiple orgasms.

The Excitement Phase

- Your Bartholin's gland secretes mucus to lubricate your vagina so your partner's penis can enter without causing friction. (See chapter 6 for information about coping with vaginal dryness.)
- Your clitoris becomes erect as it is engorged with blood.
- Your labia will probably swell.
- Your vagina may expand.
- Your skin flushes.
- Your nipples may become extra sensitive.
- Typically, your heart beats faster and your breath comes in gasps.

- Your muscle tension increases. (See chapter 9 for information about Kegel exercises, which give your vaginal muscles a workout so you can increase your pleasure and his, too.)

The Plateau Phase

- You experience continued swelling as even more blood flows to your genitals.
- In many cases, involuntary contractions of the muscles of your vagina occur.
- Your clitoris sometimes shortens and retracts under its hood.
- Your labia minora become engorged and turn reddish.
- Your heart beats still faster and your blood pressure rises.

Orgasm

- The muscles of your vagina, uterus, and anal sphincter throb rhythmically.
- Other muscles in your body may contract as well.
- Your heart rate goes up still further.

The Resolution Phase

- Blood that had engorged your pelvic region flows back to where it came from so that swelling, flushing, and muscle tension return to normal.
- You experience a profound feeling of relaxation.

HOW SEX KEEPS YOU HEALTHY AND HAPPY

Obviously, that feeling of relaxation after an orgasm is one of nature's best stress relievers. It also promotes a deep and peaceful sleep. Maybe if we all had more sex at bedtime, we would ease our national addiction to chemical sleeping pills!

Another benefit of sex is that it's good exercise. (After my husband's heart surgery, he asked his doctor when he could safely have sex again. The doctor replied that when my husband was able to climb two flights of stairs without feeling winded, he could make love with no risk. In other words, sex is as much of a workout as climbing two flights of stairs!)

In addition, all that internal activity keeps your vital functions in good shape. However, for women the actual orgasm isn't what's most important about sex. A study done by the Kinsey Institute in 2000 found that emotional health and personal relationship factors were *more important* for women's contentment with their sexual lives than achieving orgasms. In that survey, general well-being ranked as the top requirement, followed by emotional reactions during lovemaking, the attractiveness of one's partner, physical response to lovemaking, frequency of sexual activity with one's partner, the partner's sensitivity, one's own state of health, and the partner's state of health.

Putting it all together, having a wonderfully satisfying physical, emotional, and even spiritual connection to a partner during sex may just be more important to the quality of our lives than almost anything else we do. And science bears this out.

SEX REVS UP YOUR IMMUNE SYSTEM

Researchers at Wilkes University in Wilkes-Barre, Pennsylvania, studied saliva samples of a group of volunteers who reported varying frequency of sexual activity. Those with the highest frequency of sex had the most effective immune systems.

SEX IS GOOD FOR YOUR HEART

A recent report in the journal *Epidemiology and Community Health* showed that having sex several times a week reduces the likelihood of fatal heart attacks.

SEX ENHANCES YOUR SELF-ESTEEM

Researchers at the University of Texas, in an article for *Archives of Sexual Behavior*, reported that feeling good about yourself is one of the main reasons people have sex.

THE CASE FOR DO-IT-YOURSELF SEX

I will never forget when one of my patients, a wonderful woman in her seventies who was a member of the Older Women's League (OWL), gave me a catalog of sex toys. She thought I should consider sharing it with my senior patients so they could "have more fun." Good for her! But sex toys are definitely nothing new. According to a meticulously researched and critically praised 1999 book by Johns Hopkins historian Rachel P. Maines, *The Technology of Orgasm: "Hysteria," the Vibrator, and Women's Sexual Satisfaction*, vibrators were advertised as long ago as 1918 in the Sears, Roebuck catalog. The ad copy touted the device as "an aid every woman appreciates."

Farther back still, nineteenth-century doctors used to treat "hysterical" women (i.e., those who weren't getting enough sex) by manipulating their genitals. In fact, Haines writes that those doctors were the ones who welcomed the first vibrators because the devices made the job easier and shortened the patients' office visits. (And this was before managed care!)

My advice? If you grew up with taboos and myths about masturbation ("You'll go blind if you do it!" "It will make you into a crazy person!" "You'll get a terrible illness!"), train your sane and grown-up self to laugh at those threats for the fallacies they are. Masturbation is normal, in spite of the fact that Freud labeled clitoral orgasms as being "infantile." Not only that, but he also claimed that any woman who couldn't achieve what he called a "vaginal orgasm" was "frigid." As *Seattle Times* reporter Faye Flam wrote in 2005, the centennial of Freud's theory of the vaginal orgasm, "It was the idea that launched a thousand fake orgasms." In any case, Freud believed that all libido was masculine, so what did he know?

LIBIDO BOOSTERS FROM RHINOCEROS HORNS TO HORMONES

That brings me neatly to the topic you've probably been waiting for: Boosting your libido. (If you skipped right to this page, I forgive you. But promise me you'll navigate back to the beginning of the book at some point and learn all the other good stuff about your health and pleasure "down there.")

I'll get right to the point: The only true aphrodisiac for women is the male hormone testosterone. It is prescribed for some women who are postmenopausal or for some women who have had hysterectomies with ovaries removed, especially if they are young. These women have a genuine *physical* problem with arousal. I'll explain testosterone therapy in detail for those of you who need the information (skip to "Testosterone Therapy," later in this chapter, if you can't wait!), but first, about those rhinoceros horns.

The ancient Chinese are said to have ground up rhino horns and served the result as a delicacy meant to improve sexual prowess. Whether that tradition is what nearly drove the beasts to extinction is debatable, but their value as an aphrodisiac is even more dubious. The same goes for a long list of supposed passion enhancers including bananas and carrots (thought to make people feel sexy because they have a phallic appearance) and oysters (because they resemble vulvas). More recently, Marrena Lindberg, the author of *The Orgasmic Diet*, swears by dark chocolate and fish oil among other foods. Chocolate does have serotonin, which makes you feel good (that's why it's a traditional lovers' gift), but it does nothing more for your actual sex drive than any other show of affection. Fish oil, a rich source of omega-3s, has all sorts of good effects in the body, but I doubt that heavy doses will single-handedly do much for your libido.

Is Female Sexual Dysfunction the Same as Male Erectile Dysfunction?

The comparison between female sexual dysfunction (FSD) and male erectile dysfunction (ED) is disturbing to me. The word "dysfunction"—medical speak for anything that doesn't work the way it should—implies that we fully understand what is normal for women. That couldn't be further from the truth. Unlike men, who have an obvious erection and a quantifiable response (ejaculation), women have no such way to measure how things are working.

In a summary of his 1999 article entitled "The Making of a Disease," published in the *British Medical Journal,* Ray Moynihan wrote: "Researchers with close ties to drug companies are defining and classifying a new medical disorder at company sponsored meetings. The corporate sponsored definitions of 'female sexual dysfunction' are being criticized as misleading and potentially dangerous. Commonly cited prevalence estimates, which indicate that 43% of women have 'female sexual dysfunction,' are described as exaggerated and are being questioned by leading researchers."

The medicalization of female sexual dysfunction with its array of labels seems self-serving to me on the part of doctors. There is an entire section for sexual dysfunction in the American Psychiatric Association's "bible" of disorders, with codes that let physicians get paid. As far as I'm concerned, if you are not troubled by your sex life or lack of a sex life, *there is nothing wrong with you.* However, here is a list of the "definitions of sexual dysfunction," so you can assess your own situation, your needs, and your wishes—and use any of this information *only* if it makes sense to you.

Hypoactive Sexual Disorder

A deficiency or absence of sexual fantasies and desire for sexual activity. Judgment of deficiency is *made by the clinician* taking into account the person's age and the context of her life.

Female Sexual Arousal Disorder

A disorder characterized by a persistent inability to attain, or to maintain until completion of sexual activity, adequate lubrication and swelling response of sexual excitement.

Female Orgasmic Disorder

A disorder characterized by a persistent or recurrent delay or absence of orgasm after a normal excitement phase.

Then there are pheromones. In many animals other than humans, these odorless secretions somehow get the attention of potential mates, and the glands that secrete the animals' pheromones have been positively identified. Human pheromones, however, have never been shown to exist. Nonetheless, at least one smart businesswoman sells bottled pheromones for $100 per one-sixth ounce. Buyer beware.

What about Viagra? Technically, it's not a libido booster. It does nothing to get men (or women) in the mood. The little blue pill helps blood engorge the penis (but not, it seems, the clitoris), yet if a guy doesn't feel amorous in the first place, the meds won't make an erection happen. However, a recent study of women who had reduced libido as a side effect of taking antidepressants showed that the participants actually felt more interested in sex when they took Viagra.

So what's left if you want to kick it up a notch in the bedroom? The old standbys for creating a romantic ambience often do help: candlelight, soft music, and flowers. Go easy on the champagne, however. Alcohol might heighten your desire initially, but it dulls your senses if you overindulge. Ironically, birth control pills can also blunt your sex drive, but fear of pregnancy is probably an even greater turnoff so the Pill could be considered an aphrodisiac. As Jennifer Benjamin wrote in a Cosmopolitan.com article: "The July '65 issue was the first [Helen Gurley Brown] edited. 'It had a piece about the Pill, which was still new and hadn't really been written about before,' [Gurley Brown] says. 'To me, the most important thing about it was that if you weren't worried about getting pregnant, you could enjoy yourself more in bed. So we wrote a cover line to that effect.' When women saw the line—'The new pill that makes women more responsive'—they knew *exactly* what Cosmo was talking about and snatched the issue off newsstands in droves."

Finally, you could always try a hot tub. (My husband and I love ours!)

LIBIDO BUSTERS

None of those ploys for getting yourself in the mood for love will do a whole lot of good, though, if you've got a laundry list of downers in your life. Money worries, stress, fatigue, and low self-esteem can all sap your sexual energy. Also, if you have any of the medical problems "down there" that I describe in Part III of this book, then issues ranging from pain to the side effects of medication may be keeping you from being your usual lusty self. Also, depression typically makes people lose interest in sex. As I mentioned above, a recent study showed that Viagra may help depressed women feel better and have more of a sex drive, especially if they are perimenopausal.

Remember though that even if you do have libido busters in your life, the problems may well be temporary. You may also not be all that much different from most people your age when it comes to how often you have sex. Let's have a look at how the frequency of your sexual encounters compares with the average. That way you won't be torturing yourself with unrealistic standards.

HOW OFTEN IS OFTEN ENOUGH?

Most people think other people are having more sex than they are. In truth, the only people having a whole lot of sex are those in that dizzying first phase of romantic love when you are literally drugged by your own hormones and just can't keep your hands off each other. There's an old saw that goes, "Before you get married, put a bead in a big jar every time you have sex. Soon you will fill the jar. After you get married, take out a bead every time you have sex. You will never empty that jar."

Scientifically, the reason this is true is that when you move from the giddy throes of falling in love to the comfy Sunday-morning-with-pancakes-and-the-paper stage of a relationship, a different hormone takes over. You don't get a rush of adrenaline and other inner opiates that makes you crave a sexual encounter anymore. What you do get is a steady stream of the bonding hormone oxytocin. (It's the same one that pumps copiously when a woman is in labor or breastfeeding.) In other words, the neighbors probably aren't doing it any more than you are if you've been together for a while—and that's just fine.

Here is some hard data about the frequency of sexual encounters. According to a University of Chicago National Opinion Research Center General Survey in 2005, the number of reported episodes of intercourse go down with each decade of life:

- ages 18–29: a mean of 84 episodes per year
- ages 30–39: a mean of 80 episodes per year
- ages 40–49: a mean of 63.5 episodes per year
- ages 50–59: a mean of 45.8 episodes per year
- ages 60–69: a mean of 27.1 episodes per year
- ages 70 and older: a mean of 10.4 episodes per year

Frankly, I think that's good news rather than bad if you look at it this way: People in their sixties are still having sex more than twice a month and those in their seventies and beyond are making love almost once a month. Corroborating this, in the August 23, 2007 issue of the *New England Journal of Medicine,* information from the National Archive of Computerized Data on Aging (which surveyed over 3,000 men and women from the ages of fifty-seven to eighty-five) revealed that contrary to popular myth, most Americans remain sexually active into their sixties and nearly half continue to have sex regularly into their early seventies.

To be fair, however, women were significantly less likely to report being sexually active from age fifty-seven on than men were. An impressive 84 percent of men in the fifty-seven to sixty-four age group reported having some sexual contact compared with only 63 percent of women. I'm guessing this is because women are more likely to be widowed and also that women who are divorced are less likely than men to seek casual sexual encounters. In other words, the women don't have partners and the men do. (The researchers didn't ask the women about masturbation.)

Beyond that, however, the older women were more likely than their male counterparts to say that they "no longer derive much pleasure from sex." Another important finding from this detailed survey was that nearly half of the women who were sexually active reported at least one sexual problem. For example, 39 percent reported vaginal dryness and 43 percent of women reported diminished sexual desire. (Turn to chapter 6 to find out about solutions for lack of sufficient vaginal lubrication.) We'll take care of the desire issue right here, as promised, with all you need to know about testosterone therapy, which is also called androgen therapy. They mean the same thing, so let's stick with the word "testosterone."

TESTOSTERONE THERAPY

Testosterone is a male hormone, but women's adrenal glands and ovaries naturally produce some as well. In addition to playing a key role in our libido, testosterone is important for the health of many organs including bones, muscles, and even the brain. Yet our levels of testosterone decline by more than half between the ages of twenty and forty and continue to decline as we get older. Fortunately however, even when surgical removal of the ovaries robs a woman of 50 percent of what is left of her testosterone, fat cells take over to some extent just as they do for every woman. Yet for many of us, the fat cells don't supply all the testosterone we need. That's when replacement therapy is recommended.

The catch, though, is that science hasn't come up with a totally reliable test to determine the level of testosterone each of us requires to maintain a healthy sex drive and good health in general. To complicate things, many of the tissues of a woman's body, including the brain, convert testosterone into estrogen—a process known as aromatization. So is the problem really about too little estrogen and not a testosterone issue? That's a tough one, but some women who are given plenty of estrogen replacement after surgical menopause still don't feel right until a bit of testosterone is added to the mix.

Since there are no reliable blood tests to check for testosterone levels in women, simply measuring testosterone is not good enough. In most women, including women with reduced libido, the testosterone levels will show up in the normal range. But this doesn't mean there isn't a problem. Also, a big myth out there is the notion that a hair, blood, saliva, or other analysis can reliably test for testosterone. That's not true.

Even the international panel of experts that convened recently in the United States had a hard time coming up with a precise definition of testosterone insufficiency or defining how to know if a woman has insufficient testosterone. However, they suggest three basic criteria:

1. Symptoms of low testosterone should be present: unexplained fatigue, sexual function changes such as reduced libido (meaning reduced interest and pleasure in sex) and reduced sense of well-being (meaning "not feeling like your old self").

2. Because adequate estrogen is also critical to our sense of well-being and sexual function, estrogen "status" should be acceptable,

meaning if you are postmenopausal with low estrogen symptoms, you should first be treated with estrogen to see how you feel before getting a diagnosis of a low testosterone problem.

3. So-called "free testosterone" blood test results should be low, that is below or at the lowest premenopausal testosterone levels. (This is not very satisfying since, as I've already stated, the blood tests are unreliable. I guess if your levels are high, it is probably true you won't benefit from testosterone therapy, but otherwise I am not sure how meaningful blood tests are.)

The experts came up with a series of questions for doctors that can help them home in on whether you may have a problem that could benefit from testosterone therapy. Be warned, however, that there is no great body of data regarding safety and long-term effects or the best way to give testosterone to women. Yet I wanted to give you as much information as possible. Here is my version of the questions doctors are supposed to ask women. Why shouldn't you read them for yourself?

- Do you have symptoms that are typical of low testosterone, such as low libido, decreased energy, and a general sense of not feeling well?
- Is there another possible reason for these symptoms such as anemia, low thyroid, depression, or another condition? If so, get a checkup and start treatment for the other condition(s) first and see what, if any, symptoms remain.
- Is your estrogen situation okay? In other words, if you are postmenopausal with hot flashes and/or other low estrogen symptoms, or have had a hysterectomy with ovaries removed, have you tried a low dose of estrogen first to find out if that is sufficient to make you feel better? (See chapter 6, page 185 for the best way to take your dose.)
- Did you have blood testing for testosterone? Is your level low? Although blood tests are not always helpful, a low to low-normal

result may help confirm that your symptoms could be due to low testosterone.

- Did you have blood testing for sex hormone binding globulin (SHBG)?
- Are you taking oral estrogen or oral contraceptives? Oral (not transdermal, such as the patch or vaginal) estrogen can increase your sex binding proteins so your total testosterone level could be falsely elevated or normal when in fact the amount of "free" active testosterone traveling around to do its job is actually low. (See the sidebar on page 37.)

Women have been prescribed testosterone treatment for over sixty years. A synthetic testosterone called methyltestosterone was first given to women to treat their libidos and "sense of well-being." Back then the treatment was oral, but today hormone pellets or implants, skin patches or gel, are available in addition to oral forms of testosterone added to an estrogen regimen. (Testosterone is usually not taken by itself, but together with estrogen.) Research studies have shown that symptoms of reduced libido and generally feeling less than well can be helped by testosterone.

Patches of testosterone at doses of 150–300 ug/day (along with oral estrogen) have been effective but are not currently FDA-approved for use in women. The combination of oral estrogen and oral methyltestosterone at a dose of 1.25 to 2.5 mg apparently also worked in another recent study, and this combination has been around for a number of years. It is the only available prescription treatment for women in the United States. Because there are no long-term randomized controlled studies, judging its effectiveness—not to mention its safety—is difficult. However, a British study published in the *New England Journal of Medicine* in 2008 reported that a testosterone patch can boost libido in postmenopausal women. Of the 814 participants with low sexual desire, some got 300 micrograms of testosterone every day, a second group got 150 micrograms of testosterone per day, and a control group

What's the Difference between Free and Total Testosterone?

Hormones travel in the blood aboard "trains" that move them from place to place in the body. The trains are special proteins. Those called sex binding globulins are like boxcars that carry hormones rapidly from here to there. If all the testosterone in the body is on the train (that is, attached to the sex binding globulins), none is "free," meaning off the train and able to do its work. When the testosterone is riding the train, it's not performing any function in the body.

Using hormones, whether for menopausal symptoms or birth control, increases the number of "boxcars" available for testosterone, so whatever testosterone you have hops onboard, leaving none free to circulate on its own and do its job. Consequently the total testosterone level in the body may be high, but it's all taking a trip on the train rather than reporting to work.

This is why many women need to reduce rather than raise estrogen dosages and/or take a small amount of testosterone with the estrogen if libido is a big issue. What's also interesting is that as more women continue to take low-dose birth control pills up until the time of menopause (to control bleeding and to treat perimenopause symptoms as well as prevent pregnancy) they have no clue that the Pill could diminish their libido and that this could last for some time even after they stop taking the Pill.

got a placebo. The women who received the higher dose of testosterone reported having good sex two or more times a month while the placebo group had sex less than once a month. Women on the lower-dose patch said they had increased desire but the number of times they had sex didn't change. The downside, though, is that the women on the high dose of testosterone were more likely to report the growth of facial and body hair, loss of hair on the head, and lowered voices. Also, four cases of breast cancer were diagnosed among women taking testosterone compared with none among the placebo group but one of the women with breast cancer appeared to have had the disease before she started the study.

For the record, I always resist prescribing oral testosterone because I'm afraid there will be too many androgenic (male) side effects, such as lowering of good cholesterol, raising red blood count, adverse effects to the liver, and the appearance of male characteristics such as hair growth on the face and body and a low voice.

While the injectable form of testosterone is occasionally prescribed, I think it gives levels of the hormone that are too high and too unpredictable. Some women prefer pellets of testosterone injected. They last four to six months.

I am not recommending any specific testosterone regimen. However, if I were to prescribe anything, I would opt for the transdermal (meaning "through the skin") cream or patch and not an injectable and definitely not an oral one that must pass through the liver—meaning that there would be a greater effect on the liver as well as the need for a higher dose. For men, there is a commercially available testosterone gel and also an "under the tongue" pill. However, no such ready-made products are available yet for women except creams made by compounding pharmacies. (One would think science would be much more advanced when it comes to testosterone treatment in women since one-third of women have a hysterectomy and all of us will go through menopause at some point.)

However, while menopause may dampen your desire somewhat due to reduced hormone production, it does not necessarily mean the end of your sex life. If you do remain sexually active well into your postmenopausal years, you must never stop being vigilant regarding the downside of intercourse: the potential for "catching something." Only fertile women are at risk for unplanned pregnancies, but women of all ages need protection against what I like to call "sexually transmitted infections" or STIs. (The more common term is sexually transmitted diseases, or STDs.) A big part of Sex Smarts is understanding everything about STIs. So here goes:

SEXUALLY TRANSMITTED INFECTIONS (STIs)

Perhaps you are thinking that the information in this section doesn't apply to you. Maybe you are happily married, you can't imagine anything ever happening to your partner, and you assume there will never be a new man or men in your life. You may also assume that the man you love so much will never stray. I hope you're right, on all counts. But as Nora Ephron once wrote: "If you want monogamy, marry a swan." And of course, even the most faithful of spouses could leave you a widow. Life happens.

Not long ago, a divorced friend of mine called to ask sheepishly what she needed to consider before having sex with a new male friend. She wanted to be prepared but had no idea what to be worried about or what to do. She also confessed that she and her former husband—her high school sweetheart whom she married very young—had never used condoms. She had used the Pill for birth control but the issue of protection against STIs was beyond her ken.

There are plenty of women like her—maybe even you. So please read on. What you'll learn will help you whether you're a teenager just embarking on sex, a baby boomer with grandchildren who are already teens themselves, or any age in between those two. In fact, you might consider a "girls' night in" with all the generations of women in your family taking turns reading this section aloud to each other. The idea is to start a tradition that breaks the centuries-old silence women have kept about STIs. Knowledge, as they say, is power. Share it with those you love.

HOW NOT TO GET STIs

The only sure way to avoid getting a sexually transmitted disease is not to have sex. Obviously, the same goes for avoiding getting pregnant. That being so, proponents of so-called "abstinence-only sex education" want to limit your "education" to one mandate: "Don't do it." What planet do they live on?

Okay, sometimes the abstinence-only folks also deign to give you scary statistics about the failure rate of various methods of practicing "safe sex." But they insist that teaching people about how to protect themselves from catching STIs (or getting pregnant) encourages sexual activity. I am definitely not in that camp. Human nature is what encourages sexual activity. In fact a study from the Johns Hopkins Bloomberg School of Public Health that was released on December 29, 2008 showed that teens who promise to remain abstinent until marriage are just as likely to have premarital sex as are teens who don't make that promise. Not only that, but the abstinence-only teens are statistically far less likely to use condoms and are therefore at greater risk of getting pregnant and contracting STIs.

As you know by now, the essence of my philosophy about health in general and sexual health in particular is that you deserve to be the one who's in charge. In order for that to happen, you need complete and easy-to-understand information. That's why I not only dismiss the abstinence-only mandate but I also go beyond the notion of "safe sex." Living has risks. The more fully and joyfully you live, the more risks you face. Anyway, as I've already pointed out (see "How Sex Keeps You Healthy and Happy" earlier in this chapter), sex can actually be good for your health.

Consequently, I coined the term Smart Sex. That means:

- Not sleeping with just anyone you meet. You wouldn't buy a new car without knowing what features it offers. Doesn't it also make sense to get to know the person you're about to swap germs with?

Can I Catch STIs or Get Pregnant from Toilet Seats?

Let me dispel a decades-old myth. When I entered nursing school way back in 1967, the head nurse advised us girls (our class was all "girls" in those days) to beware of toilet seats. "When it comes to getting pregnant," she warned, "you never know how close is too close." She further explained that toilet seats might contain the "seeds" to start a pregnancy. She was wrong, but we believed her. And back then it never entered our minds that we might get an STI from a toilet seat. Pregnancy was the big scare when it came to messing around with boys or sitting on wet toilet seats. Today, when women get an unusual rash "down there," they may worry that they got the infection from a dirty public toilet seat. Trust me, that's virtually impossible. Viruses can't live very long outside the body. I have *never* seen a study reporting any toilet-seat-related disease.

You can use those paper toilet seat covers if they make you feel better or you can lift up the seat and "hover" if you're good at it, but personally I just sit down. For obvious reasons, I wipe off a wet seat but I rarely try to balance myself in that "squat and hang" position, especially not in the bathroom of a moving airplane or train. As you know if you've tried that, one lurch of the vehicle can mean that you're guaranteed to miss your mark. My advice is wipe it down, sit, and be comfortable.

- Practicing "Emotional Smart Sex." Is your partner married to someone else? Is he abusive? Does he cheat? Does he ask you to do things that are painful or uncomfortable? If so, you are putting your emotional self at risk. If your girlfriend had a partner like that, what would you say to her? Smart Sex protects your heart and spirit as well as your body.

How Do I Buy and Use Condoms?

You need this information whether you're a teenager contemplating your first sexual encounter or a suddenly single senior getting back into the dating scene, or anybody in between. As one of my divorced patients said when she asked me for advice before taking a new relationship to the romance level, "The only time I ever handled a condom was when I fished one out of the pocket of my teenage son's jeans before doing the laundry!"

Condoms are regulated as medical devices and are subject to random sampling and testing by the Food and Drug Administration. Each latex condom manufactured in the United States is tested electronically for holes before packaging. The failure of latex condoms to protect against STIs (or pregnancy) usually results from inconsistent or incorrect use rather than condom breakage or holes.

Condoms made of materials other than latex are available, but some of them have higher breakage and slippage rates when compared with latex condoms, and all of them are usually more costly than latex. The two general categories of non-latex condoms are:

1. Those made of polyurethane or other synthetic materials. They provide protection against STIs and pregnancy equal to that of latex condoms. These are a good choice for people who have a latex allergy.

2. The so-called "natural membrane condoms." These are often incorrectly referred to as "lambskin condoms." They are usually made from lamb cecum (part of the large intestine) and can have holes or "pores." These pores do not allow the passage of sperm, but they are more than ten times the diameter of some sexually transmitted viruses including HIV. Laboratory studies have shown that viral STI transmission can occur with

natural membrane condoms. In other words, they don't prevent STIs.

Here are my recommendations to ensure the proper use of condoms:

- Carefully handle the condom to avoid damaging it.
- Wait until your partner's penis is erect before one or both of you puts the condom on his penis.
- Don't have any genital contact until the condom is in place.
- Ensure adequate vaginal lubrication during sex by using water-based lubricants if necessary. (This is especially important for postmenopausal women who have much less natural lubrication.)
- Use only water-based lubricants such as K-Y Jelly with latex condoms. Oil-based lubricants such as petroleum jelly, massage oils, body lotions, and cooking oil can weaken latex.
- Have your partner withdraw while his penis is still erect, meaning right after he ejaculates. Don't wait until it's too late, when he is flaccid and the condom falls off inside.
- Have your partner hold the condom firmly against the base of his penis during withdrawal.
- If you engage in sexual activity involving more than one body part during any given sexual encounter, use a different condom for each type of intercourse, whether vaginal, oral, or anal.
- You may also want to consider using a female condom. This is a plastic pouch that is inserted into the vagina. It is an effective mechanical barrier to viruses, including HIV, and to semen. However, female condoms cost a lot more than male condoms.

- Using birth control. (See chapter 5, pages 140–57.)
- Asking potential partners to bring a medical history, including tests they've had, what I call the "Smart Sex Seal of Approval."

- In particular, making sure potential partners have been screened for the human immunodeficiency virus (HIV), which can cause an infection that can lead to acquired immunodeficiency syndrome (AIDS). Getting the results of an HIV test takes only a few days, but if your potential partner was recently exposed to the virus, he may not test positive for up to six weeks or more depending on the type of test used. Don't take his word for the fact that he hasn't just been with someone else. Have him wait to take the test until six or more weeks have gone by and resist getting physical until his test result is negative. (If he's not willing to hold off for that long, he's not going to be a keeper anyway!)
- Having condoms at the ready—even if you're postmenopausal and not worried about contraception. Condoms protect you against viruses that love to grow in mucous membranes. (Diaphragms and vaginal spermicides do *not* protect against viral STIs.)

VIRAL SEXUALLY TRANSMITTED INFECTIONS

There are two types of STIs: those caused by viruses and those caused by bacteria. I'm going to teach you first about the viral STIs. When you contract a virus, it might disappear on its own after one or two years and you'll never even know you had it. Or the virus could remain dormant for years and then suddenly cause symptoms. What's more, if your immune system doesn't fight off the virus by itself, no antibiotic or "antiviral" drug can eliminate it. However, viruses can be managed so that you can live long and well—and continue to enjoy sex—in spite of them.

Human Papilloma Virus (HPV)

There are over one hundred strains of HPV in all. Of those, thirty-five strains can infect the genitals. The rest can cause warts on other surface/skin areas of the body such as the feet (plantar warts) and the hands. What we're concerned with here are the strains that can infect the genitals. Of those thirty-five strains, some (especially strains 6 and 11) can cause genital warts (see "HPV and Genital Warts" later in this chapter). The remaining fifteen strains can cause abnormalities that could eventually lead to cervical cancer unless they are detected early enough by a Pap smear (see below). These strains can also cause oral and anal cancer. Virus strains 16 and 18 pose the highest risk for cancer.

This information is relatively new. For decades, early detection of cervical cancer as a result of a Pap smear was all that medicine had to offer women. However, years before we knew what caused cervical cancer, research showed that celibate nuns simply do not get cervical cancer whereas sex workers have a particularly high risk. The problem with the "nuns versus frequent sex" research is that it suggested that you had to have had multiple sex partners in order to get cervical cancer. Not true. A woman can get HPV that potentially leads to cervical cancer after a single sexual experience. For that matter, she can get it from her husband if he's cheating. An estimated 85 percent of women who have ever been sexually active will be exposed to genital HPV during their lifetimes.

The good news is that for over ninety out of one hundred women who get infected, the virus simply disappears on its own after twelve to twenty-four months once the immune system kicks in. For the remaining women, the virus "persists." If that happens to you, you may be at risk for cell changes and eventually for cervical cancer.

The Pap Test

If you have ever had sex at all—even once or even with only one man in your lifetime—you should have a regular Pap test or "cervical smear." Of course the recommendation doesn't apply if your cervix has been removed because you had a hysterectomy. (Not all types of hysterectomies remove the cervix, and I've treated patients who didn't know what type of hysterectomy they had. See chapter 7 for clarification.)

Even if you are sixty-five or older and your doctor says you can stop having your regular Pap test, you may be putting yourself at risk. The

TEST	RESULT	LIMITS	LAB
GYN REPORT			RJ
TEST ORDERED:			
192005 MONOLAYER LIQUID BASED PREP			
Number of Slides = 1			RJ
SOURCE:			
CERVIX			
ENDOCERVICAL			RJ
CLINICAL HISTORY:			
455.6 ; UNSPECIFIED HEMORRHOIDS WITHOUT MENTION OF COMPLICATION			
424.0 ; MITRAL VALVE DISORDERS			
715.90 ; OSTEOARTHROSIS, UNSPECIFIED WHETHER GENERALIZED OR LOCALIZED,			S
			RJ

```
****************************************************************
DIAGNOSIS:
NEGATIVE FOR INTRAEPITHELIAL LESION AND MALIGNANCY.
```

| | | | RJ |

```
SPECIMEN ADEQUACY:
SATISFACTORY FOR EVALUATION. ENDOCERVICAL AND/OR SQUAMOUS METAPLASTIC
CELLS (ENDOCERVICAL COMPONENT) ARE PRESENT.
****************************************************************
```

			MF
PERFORMED BY:			
GYNECOLOGIC MONO-LAYER PAP			RN

```
THE PAP SMEAR IS A SCREENING TEST DESIGNED TO AID IN THE DETECTION
OF PREMALIGNANT AND MALIGNANT CONDITIONS OF THE UTERINE CERVIX. IT
IS NOT A DIAGNOSTIC PROCEDURE AND SHOULD NOT BE USED AS THE SOLE
MEANS OF DETECTING CERVICAL CANCER. BOTH FALSE-POSITIVE AND FALSE-
NEGATIVE REPORTS DO OCCUR.
```

Pap smear test results

tacit assumption your doctor is making is that if you were going to get cervical cancer from a latent HPV infection, you'd have gotten it by now. Beyond that, the doctor is assuming that you're no longer sexually active. If you know better, even if you're in a monogamous relationship and especially if you're not, get your Pap test! (For the record, the name of the test isn't short for "Papilloma." It's short for the name of one of its inventors, Dr. Georgios Papanikolaou.)

The Test for HPV

In terms of prevention and early detection, we now have something more than just the Pap smear. Did you know there is a test for the presence of HPV in the transformation zone of your cervix where the virus likes to grow and cause cell changes? The HPV test checks for the high-risk strains of the virus that could cause cervical cancer. The test is simple and can be done at the same time as your Pap smear, and with the same brush or swab. If you find out that you carry the virus, you can be watched more closely. An HPV test is recommended as a routine preventive measure for women ages thirty and over along with the Pap test. Incidentally, testing younger women routinely for HPV doesn't help all that much because about one in four of them will test positive while their bodies are taking up to two years to successfully fight off the virus. Then it magically disappears and any future HPV test for that strain of the virus will be negative.

Some doctors don't see the need to do both tests, and because the Pap is already so well accepted, they figure why rock the boat? Actually, there's a terrific reason to flip that boat right over: cancer prevention. I remember testifying about the value of the HPV test to legislators in Illinois. One male legislator said (I'm paraphrasing here): "Why would any woman need an HPV test if she is married and in a monogamous relationship?" I asked him if his wife had regular Pap tests, and he responded that, yes, she was religious about getting them. I reminded him—as gently as my preaching nature allowed—that being religious about Pap tests amounts to being religious about getting checked for cell changes caused by HPV.

Only if you test positive on two or more occasions for the high-risk, cancer-causing strains of the virus are you at risk for cervical cancer. The multiple positive results mean that the virus didn't clear up on its on own. Either way, the HPV test gives you tremendous peace of mind. If you test positive once and then test negative, you can relax. If you test positive two or more times, you can get help before it's too late.

Women who test negative for the virus and have a normal Pap test (close to 95 percent of us will test negative for precancerous changes) only need to repeat those tests once every three years. Women who test positive for the virus should continue yearly checkups, and their doctors

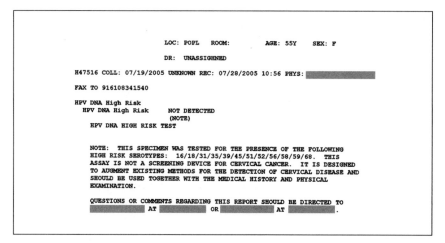

LOC: POPL   ROOM: AGE: 55Y   SEX: F

DR: UNASSIGNED

H47516 COLL: 07/19/2005 UNKNOWN REC: 07/28/2005 10:56 PHYS:

FAX TO 916108341540

HPV DNA High Risk
   HPV DNA High Risk   NOT DETECTED
                           (NOTE)
      HPV DNA HIGH RISK TEST

NOTE: THIS SPECIMEN WAS TESTED FOR THE PRESENCE OF THE FOLLOWING
HIGH RISK SEROTYPES: 16/18/31/35/39/45/51/52/56/58/59/68. THIS
ASSAY IS NOT A SCREENING DEVICE FOR CERVICAL CANCER. IT IS DESIGNED
TO AUGMENT EXISTING METHODS FOR THE DETECTION OF CERVICAL DISEASE AND
SHOULD BE USED TOGETHER WITH THE MEDICAL HISTORY AND PHYSICAL
EXAMINATION.

QUESTIONS OR COMMENTS REGARDING THIS REPORT SHOULD BE DIRECTED TO
               AT   OR   AT   .

HPV test results

can take extra measures to ensure that any possible cervical cell changes are caught early, before they turn into cancer. This usually means doing a colposcopy after dabbing a vinegar solution on the cervix. The vinegar solution makes the abnormal cells turn white. Using an instrument called a colposcope, which shines a light and magnifies the cervix, the doctor can look for cell changes that may have been missed by the Pap test. (The Pap test is far from perfect, as it requires someone to examine hundreds of cells under the microscope to detect changes.)

It's as simple as that. You have a right to know everything about your health, so ask your doctor for an HPV test at your next gynecologic exam. (See "Diagnosis and Treatment of Cervical Cancer" later in this chapter, to learn what happens next if the doctor sees abnormal cells during a colposcopy.)

The Vaccine against Cancers Caused by HPV

If the HPV test is good news, the HPV vaccine is even better news. Imagine it! We not only now know that HPV is the *only* cause of cervical cancer, we actually have a vaccine to prevent it. Hurrah! This is the first vaccine against a cancer that has a single cause. There is the hepatitis B vaccine that is given to infants to protect them against the sexually and blood-borne acquired hepatitis B virus that can not only cause infection but also liver cancer. However, hepatitis B is only one of many other causes of liver cancer. Cervical cancer is the first cancer known to be caused solely by a single agent: the high-risk strains of the HPV virus. And now we have a vaccine.

The current HPV vaccine, Gardasil, protects young women against four strains of the virus. It is recommended for girls at age eleven or twelve, but is approved for girls as young as age nine and young women up to age twenty-six. It works best if it is given before a woman becomes sexually active and is therefore exposed to the virus—which could theoretically be helpful to women much older than twenty-six. In fact, it is being studied in women up to age forty-five and so far it has been shown to be effective and safe. Women at any age could be exposed to a cancer-causing or genital-wart-causing strain of the virus with a new or unfaithful partner and deserve to be protected. However, because the vaccine has yet to been approved for older women, insurance will not pay for it.

The vaccine has the potential to protect women from cervical cancer caused by the two strains of HPV that are responsible for 70 percent of the cases of HPV-caused cancers. In addition, Gardasil protects against the two strains of HPV that cause 90 percent of the cases of genital warts. Research suggests that the vaccine may also be partially effective against up to ten other strains of HPV, so the overall reduction in cancer risk may be even greater than originally expected.

Incidentally, Gardasil may also protect against anal cancer and oral pharyngeal cancers in both men and women. The latter two forms, typically caused by smoking and excessive alcohol use, are now increasingly caused by high-risk HPV strains resulting from oral sex. Anal cancer, most often caused by HPV, can result from vaginal sex as well as anal sex. The virus can infect all the surrounding genital tissue. The vaccine also protects against vulvar and vaginal dysplasia and cancer caused by the high-risk strains of HPV. The maker of the vaccine is hoping to get approval for the vaccine for boys, too, by 2009 when data are all in.

As this book goes to press, another vaccine, Cervarix, is awaiting approval from the FDA. This vaccine will be cancer-fighting only as it will protect against HPV 16 and 18; it will not protect against genital warts. Which vaccine is best and which will last longest to protect women from cancer will not be known until years of research have been done.

However, there's no need to wait years to protect girls and young women from cervical cancer as well as oral and anal cancer. We've got Gardasil right now, and it's been tested in more than five years of clinical trials. We do need more long-term research regarding the vaccine's safety and efficacy, but take comfort in the fact that the material in Gardasil is very similar to the material in the hepatitis B vaccine, which we give to infants without concern.

So now that we have the vaccine, there must be a line around the block to sign up, right? Unfortunately not. The advertisements are compelling, with girls and young women claiming their right to be protected against HPV. But the marketing campaign does not seem to be effective. There are people who are reluctant to have their daughters vaccinated, mainly because of the "nun versus sex worker" idea, meaning that their daughter is "good" and therefore won't get HPV. The other common argument is that getting the vaccine will somehow encourage young women to have sex—as though the threat of HPV were the only thing holding them back!

These statements make me crazy. It sounds as if parents are saying they are more worried about their daughters having sex (inevitable eventually, even years down the line) than they are about protecting them from cancer! Even if a woman remains celibate until marriage, the truth is that she'll never know exactly where her husband's penis has been. Even seemingly "nice boys" can carry the risky strains of HPV and pass them on to their wives. Men don't wear flashing "I Carry HPV" signs and there is no effective HPV test for men to see if they do carry it. Plus, to state a blunt reality, there is the possibility of rape—by a date or a stranger. Statistics show that one in three women are raped or have sex against their will, and their rapists may carry STIs, including HPV.

The bottom line for mothers, grandmothers, and daughters to consider is this: We are *all* at risk for HPV infection as a result of being lively, healthy human beings. The vaccine does the most good when it is administered before a girl or woman's "sexual debut." It is considered safe and, as I said, it is not dissimilar to the hepatitis B vaccine we give our infants. It's been tested on thousands of girls and young women who have been carefully monitored for more than five years. As of 2009, over thirty million doses have been given, and the worst confirmed side effects of the vaccine are a painful injection site and risk of fainting from the shot itself. Of course, monitoring any girl or woman who gets the vaccine is to be advised, but given the known safety of the vaccine so far and the known risk of HPV, protecting women appears to be a wise choice.

The window of opportunity for our daughters is very small. Every mother needs to ask herself one question: If you choose not to give your daughter the vaccine and she contracts cervical cancer some day, or suffers from infertility from treatment of HPV cell changes on her cervix, could you live with your decision? "If only . . ." are very painful words, especially when it comes to conditions as serious as cancer and infertility.

Diagnosis and Treatment of Cervical Cancer

If your Pap test shows abnormal cells and/or you test positive for HPV on two or more HPV tests in a row, your doctor will perform a colposcopy to look for the abnormal cells (see "The Test for HPV" above). The next step is a biopsy of those areas, which means excising a small amount of tissue to be sent to a laboratory for testing. In a week or so, you'll get the results with a report of cell changes, called dysplasia or cervical intraepithelial neoplasia (CIN), classified according to degree as follows:

- CIN 1 means you have an active HPV infection that your body has not yet fought off although it is almost certainly in the process of trying. There is no treatment needed at this point. The best course is what we call "watchful waiting." Years ago doctors used to recommend excising cells at this early stage. We now know that the treatment is far too aggressive for CIN 1 and that it unnecessarily puts women at risk for complications in subsequent pregnancies. All you need to do is have another Pap smear in six months to find out if the situation has resolved itself—which is almost always the case.
- CIN 2 and 3 are usually lumped together as they can be hard to differentiate. These are precancerous lesions. The only way to get rid of them is to remove the transformation zone or "donut hole area" (see chapter 1, page 11), where HPV loves to grow. The cells will be removed in one of the following ways:

  1. **Cryosurgery:** This is an office procedure performed while you are lying on your back with your feet in the stirrups as for a pelvic exam (see chapter 3, page 99). The procedure doesn't hurt, although you may feel a little cramping. You don't need any anesthesia. Tubelike instruments called cryoprobes are inserted into your vagina so that they cover the abnormal cervical tissue, i.e., the transformation zone. Liquid nitrogen flows through the metal tubes and freezes them. The procedure is then repeated at a three-minute interval. This destroys the abnormal tissue.
  2. **Loop electrosurgical excision procedure (LEEP):** This can be an office procedure or it can be done at a hospital as an out-patient procedure (meaning you don't have to stay overnight). Again you lie on your back and put your feet in the stirrups, as

for a pelvic exam. You'll be given an anesthetic called a cervical block that numbs the cervix. A low-voltage electrical wire is inserted to excise the abnormal tissue. You should be back to your normal activity level in one to three days, although sex and the use of tampons should be avoided for three weeks.

3. **Cone biopsy:** The name derives from the cone-shaped section of the cervix, which is removed. It contains the "transformation zone" where HPV loves to settle in and multiply. A small amount of tissue surrounding this area is also removed in hopes of getting what is called a "clean margin" of normal cells. (If the margin is "clean," your test result is "negative," which is good news even though it sounds bad. Confusing, I know!) A cone biopsy is most often an out-patient procedure, meaning that you don't have to stay overnight in the hospital. You'll either get an epidural to numb the genital area or you'll get general anesthesia. Most women are back to normal activities within one week after the procedure. The tissue that is removed is examined under a microscope. A cone biopsy may cause complications in future pregnancies such as an incompetent cervix that doesn't stay closed tightly enough for you to carry a pregnancy to full term unless you get a "stitch," meaning that a surgeon sews your cervix closed and then removes the surgical thread when you're ready to deliver. However, even LEEP may cause this problem. Also, the stitch almost always works and some women don't even need one.

- CIN 4 is carcinoma in situ, which is "Stage 0" right before the cells become cancerous. At this point the cells are still in situ (Latin for "in place") and have not yet penetrated what is called the "basement membrane" so that they can pass through and make their way to other parts of the body. A cone biopsy is required but you'll probably need no further treatment. However,

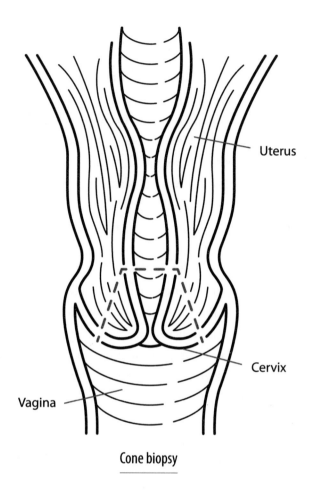

Uterus

Cervix

Vagina

Cone biopsy

your doctor may recommend a hysterectomy "just in case." If you want to get pregnant, a hysterectomy is obviously not an option you're going to want to choose. Women's body parts are so often treated as potential time bombs for cancer and the prevailing philosophy tends to be that you might as well just take them out. Don't be too quick to fall for that. Get a second opinion before you agree to lose your uterus. (See chapter 7 for a complete explanation of hysterectomies.).

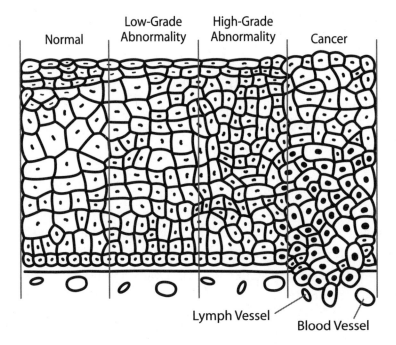

Changes in cervical cells

If your test results show that you have one of the four stages of cancer, you need to see a cancer specialist, called an oncologist.

HPV and Genital Warts

About 90 percent of genital warts are caused by the HPV 6 and 11 "low-risk" strains of HPV and many of us will get infected at some point. As we've already seen, these strains do not cause cancer. The other good news about HPV 6 and 11 infections is two-fold:

- They are often asymptomatic.
- Even if warts do occur, typically three to six months after exposure, they usually go away on their own after your immune system wins the battle—but this can take months or even years.

The bad news, however, is three-fold:

- If they're symptomatic, genital warts—depending on size and location— are unsightly, can bleed easily, and can be painful and itchy.
- They are very infectious.
- They can be very hard to treat.

Diagnosis of Genital Warts

Genital warts are usually flat or raised growths anywhere around the genital area. They can occur on the cervix and in the vagina, urethra, and anus. If you notice growths of this description, see your doctor. She can usually make the diagnosis of genital warts simply by looking at your tissues, but a biopsy is needed if:

- the lesions do not respond to standard therapy
- the disease worsens during therapy
- the patient has a chronic immune deficiency
- the warts are unusual in appearance, including being pigmented, hard, or ulcerated

Treatment of Genital Warts

An asymptomatic HPV 6 or 11 infection may sometimes be diagnosed as a result of a routine Pap smear. Mild cell changes referred to as ASCUS or LSIL is what you will see on the report of your Pap test. The result of your HPV test (if you have one done) will show none of the high-risk cancer strains. While no treatment is necessary, you are capable of infecting your partner until the infection subsides on its own, which may take many months. If your Pap test is abnormal, then you will need a Pap smear in six months to find out whether or not these cell changes—signs of HPV infection—are gone.

As for visible warts, there is no clear-cut evidence that any of the available treatments are superior to any other and no single treatment is ideal for all patients or all warts. Because genital warts may eventually go away on their own, some people forego treatment. In fact, internationally famous Australian HPV expert Dr. Ian Fraser maintains that ideally genital warts should not be treated. He believes the irritation and inflammation from treatment simply delay the body's own resolution of the problem and spread the virus further. However, please remember that you need to avoid sex with a new partner until genital warts either go away on their own or are treated. Your current partner likely already has the same type of virus and his body may have already fought it off. You can use a condom as a precaution but remember that the infection may involve areas of your genitals that are not covered by a condom.

The primary goal of treating genital warts is to remove what is visible in order to lessen the possibility of spreading or shedding of the virus to a partner. Treatment may also reduce the actual HPV infection, but it does not eliminate it. Again, you remain infectious until your immune system kicks in and fights off that strain—hopefully for good. The jury is still out regarding whether the same strain can reinfect you, but other strains can infect you in the future so precautions are always worth taking.

If you choose to be treated, you may require a course of therapy rather than a single treatment. Should one method of treatment fail to work, your doctor will switch to another method. The majority of genital warts respond within three months of therapy.

There are two treatment regimens, which are divided into "patient-applied" and "practitioner-applied" methods. I have found that many patients prefer to treat themselves because this means they don't have to miss work for doctor's appointments.

Patient-applied treatments (prescriptions from your doctor are necessary):

- Podofilox 0.5 percent solution or gel applied to visible genital warts twice a day for three days, followed by four days of no therapy. This cycle may be repeated, as necessary, for up to four cycles.

- Imiquimod 5 percent cream. Patients should apply imiquimod cream once daily at bedtime, three times a week for up to sixteen weeks. The treatment area should be washed with soap and water six to ten hours after the application.

Practitioner-administered treatments:

- Cryotherapy ("freezing") using liquid nitrogen or a special machine. This may need to be repeated every one or two weeks until the warts are gone.
- Podophyllin resin 10 to 25 percent in a compound tincture of benzoin. This is a much stronger dose than what you would use at home. The treatment can be repeated weekly if necessary. Some physicians, myself included, suggest that the preparation should be thoroughly washed off one to four hours after application to reduce local irritation. There have been rare case reports of severe systemic effects from podophyllin, but overall, the treatment is very safe.
- Trichloroacetic acid (TCA) or bichloroacetic acid (BCA) 80 to 90 percent. This topical treatment is applied with a cotton swab and can be repeated weekly if necessary.
- Surgical removal either by scraping or shaving the warts or by electrocautery with a special machine.

HERPES SIMPLEX VIRUS OR HSV

There are two types of herpes simplex virus: HSV-1 and HSV-2. Oral herpes, or HSV-1, causes "cold sores" or "fever blisters," usually on the lips or in the mouth. Genital herpes, or HSV-2, causes blisters in the genital area and on the buttocks and anus. Although you can occasionally develop genital herpes by having oral sex with someone who has HSV-1, a genital infection with HSV-1 is much less likely to come back than an HSV-2 infection is. HSV-2 is transmitted sexually. HSV-1 can be acquired from any direct contact, even touch, and is thus not considered an STI. In the days before all health-care workers wore latex gloves, a patient with a cold sore could infect the finger of a dentist who could then pass it on to other patients.

Once HSV-2 finds a hospitable environment, meaning a mucous membrane, the virus burrows in and lives in the nerve endings of the tissue forever. You can never get rid of the virus altogether, even with antiviral medication, but at least the attacks and the pain can be minimized. HSV generally lies dormant most of the time, with only periodic flare-ups. These active episodes almost always diminish eventually and in some people they stop altogether. Many women experience flares in response to stress and during their menstrual periods, but current medications can minimize or suppress this frequency and severity.

The HSV-2 virus can be "silent" for years before a first episode of blisters occurs. It is estimated that more than 20 percent of adults are infected with HSV-2 and there are up to one million first-time infections per year. Most people infected with HSV-2 do not know they have been infected. They may have mild or unrecognized infections but shed the virus intermittently in the genital area without realizing it. However, they are infectious and can spread the disease even without visible ulcers or skin lesions.

A first-time or primary outbreak of herpes means your immune system has not previously been exposed to the virus and so it has no antibodies to protect you. As a result, the symptoms can range from almost nothing at all to severe, as in the case of one forty-four-year-old patient of mine I remember well. She came to me complaining of horrendous vulvar pain and difficulty urinating. She was in severe distress and had no idea what was wrong with her. When I asked what was new or different in her life, she said that she had gone through a difficult divorce but that she had recently met a wonderful man and had started a sexual relationship with him. I knew immediately what was probably going on. She had the usual symptoms of an HSV-2 infection.

Symptoms of HSV-2

- pain in the genital area and/or the anal area
- difficulty urinating
- blisters in the genital and/or anal area

The typical initial outbreak lasts about two to three weeks while your body forms antibodies to help fight off the infection. Once you have the antibodies, the symptoms of subsequent infections are less severe, shorter in duration, and may cover a smaller area of your vulva and vagina or anus. (HSV-2 antibodies are different from HSV-1 antibodies, although to some degree they overlap and can help fight both types of herpes infections). Researchers believe that most genital occurrences of the viral infection after the first one go unnoticed. Remember though: That doesn't mean the virus can't be passed to a partner. Up to one-third of women may have HSV on the cervix when they have an asymptomatic occurrence. They could pass the HSV on to a partner and not know it. Cervix lesions don't hurt, so you wouldn't know you have them.

Also, some people who have been exposed to HSV by a sexual partner before they get married to someone else may not have their first noticeable occurrence for twenty or thirty years or more. This is obviously a potential cause for mistrust in stable monogamous relationships unless both partners understand how long the virus can be dormant.

Other people may have recurrences of HSV-2 as often as four to six times a year.

Sometimes the outbreaks occur in the anus even if no anal sex occurred. The entire genital area is supplied by the nerves that carry the virus.

Diagnosing Genital Herpes

Your doctor can use a combination of a thorough medical history, a physical exam (the least reliable), a viral culture or "swab," and blood tests to make the precise diagnosis. Keeping an accurate health journal (see chapter 3) will help your doctor. Note in your journal the dates of outbreaks and any possible "triggers" such as stressful events associated with outbreaks. Also note sexual activity and your symptoms.

Your doctor will do a pelvic exam. This can be difficult and painful, especially for a first-time infection. In addition to checking for blisters, your doctor will examine the lymph nodes in your groin, which can get swollen and tender. Doctors mistakenly diagnose symptoms as herpes up to 20 percent of the time, so cultures can be a big help to be sure.

To culture the virus, a non-cotton swab is rubbed over the ulcer base or skin that looks abnormal. The resulting specimen is placed in a vial containing liquid, and it is then sent to a laboratory. If the culture is positive, you are almost 100 percent certain the diagnosis is correct. However, viral culture has a sensitivity of only 50 percent, meaning that even if herpes is present, the culture will only come back positive 50 percent of the time. This happens more often in patients with recurrent infections or with healing lesions because the virus is somehow missed and not scraped onto the swab.

In the case of a negative test result, blood tests are useful in confirming a clinical diagnosis of genital herpes. The Western blot blood test is considered the gold standard and is almost 100 percent accurate. There are almost no false positive or negative results. It is spot-on.

Routine testing of people over the age of twenty-five who have no symptoms is discouraged because the prevalence of positive antibody results for HSV-2 is known to be high and also because therapy would not be indicated anyway. Not only that, but diagnosis can be extremely upsetting, and it serves no purpose.

I mentioned that a physical exam is the least reliable diagnostic tool for HSV-2. Even so, the blisters and ulcerations I saw surrounding the labia and urethra of the forty-four-year-old patient I mentioned earlier were almost certainly from a primary (first time ever) outbreak of an HSV-2 infection. Her painful and difficult urination was caused by multiple blisters surrounding and inside her urethra. Sure enough, six days later a culture of the fluid from one of the blisters came back positive for HSV-2. Fortunately, my patient's symptoms had been relieved by the only antiviral medication available for HSV at the time, acyclovir. (I had prescribed it right away rather than make her wait in agony for the test results since it's safe and I was pretty certain of the diagnosis.) I say "fortunately" because sometimes a primary HSV-2 infection involving the urethra can be so severe that urination is almost completely blocked due to the ballooning blisters. Hospitalization and a urethral catheter are temporarily necessary.

Treatment of HSV-2

When I first started practicing medicine in the late 1970s, there was no effective treatment for HSV-2 except symptomatic relief with Blistex and other non-curative ointments for lips, and sometimes the amino acid lysine. Soon, however, a topical form of Zovirax became available. It wasn't really effective yet but it made doctors like me feel as though we were doing *something* for this annoying and painful condition. Today there are three very effective choices of oral (systemic) medications available. The major differences among them are the cost, whether your insurance covers the one your doctor prescribes, and how many pills you need to take. These medications target only the virus and don't attack the healthy bacteria in your body. Systemic antiviral medications—as opposed to the minimally effective antiviral topical creams—partially control the symptoms and signs of a first herpes episode and treat recurrent episodes well. They also work when used as daily therapy to prevent episodes from coming back. However, these drugs neither get rid of the virus altogether nor affect the risk, frequency, or severity of recurrences after the drug is discontinued. Here are the drugs:

- Zovirax (acyclovir)
- Valtrex (valacyclovir)
- Famvir (famciclovir)

Some Things I Tell My Patients about HSV-2

- If this is your first episode of genital herpes, you should know that suppressive and episodic antiviral therapies are available. They're effective in preventing or shortening the duration of recurrent episodes.
- You should let your current partner know that you have genital herpes and tell future partners before initiating a sexual relationship.
- You can transmit HSV even if you don't have symptoms.
- Asymptomatic viral shedding is more frequent in genital HSV-2 infection than in the much less common genital HSV-1 infection and is most frequent in the first twelve months after acquiring HSV-2.
- Between flare-ups, latex condoms can reduce your risk of getting HSV-2 from a male partner. However, the condom won't protect him from contracting HSV-2 from you.
- You should abstain from sexual activity when blisters or warning (prodromal) symptoms are present.

These three drugs work by stopping the duplication and shedding of the virus from body cells. They are all similar in action, varying primarily in the dosage and timing. The sooner you start taking one of the medications when you begin having symptoms, the better it works. Famvir is unique. A recent study showed that a single one-day dose of 1,000 mg (four tablets) can be taken twice, starting within six hours of symptoms, and that's it. The other regimens suggest treatment for three to five days depending on the dosage.

Effective episodic treatment of recurrent herpes requires beginning the medication within one day of lesion onset, or during the "prodromal" or warning symptoms such as tingling or pain that precedes some outbreaks. Ask your doctor to give you a prescription for the medication with instructions on how to begin treatment immediately when symptoms begin.

What works:

- Acyclovir 400 mg orally three times a day for five days
- Acyclovir 800 mg orally twice a day for five days
- Famciclovir 125 mg orally twice a day for five days
- Valacyclovir 500 mg orally twice a day for three to five days
- Valacyclovir 1.0 g orally once a day for five days

Suppressive therapy reduces the frequency of genital herpes recurrences by 70 to 80 percent among people who have had frequent recurrences, for example six recurrences per year. Many people treated with suppressive therapy report no symptomatic outbreaks at all. Treatment is probably also effective in people with less frequent recurrences although the research is not as conclusive.

The frequency of recurrent outbreaks naturally diminishes over time, so every so often you should ask your doctor to reassess the need for continued therapy.

This treatment helps reduce the virus's ability to spread to your partner but does not completely eliminate this process. The same three drugs listed above are the best choices for suppressive therapy. Fortunately, side effects and allergic reactions to these antiviral medications are rare.

Remember the patient I told you about with the painful first-time HSV-2 outbreak? She was devastated by the diagnosis of HSV-2 and by the realization that she was at lifelong risk for recurrences. I assured her that episodes tend to get less frequent over time, and sometimes stop altogether. Yet how could she have prevented this infection in the first place? Having her new partner use a condom would have been smart, although a condom doesn't protect completely against the HSV virus because it can live in the cells outside the prophylactic's coverage zone. I asked why she hadn't had an honest discussion with her new partner about each other's prior sexual history and infections. She admitted that she didn't want to offend him or act as though she didn't trust him. How crazy is that? Crazier still, why didn't he tell her that he had herpes if he knew? Perhaps he was embarrassed or perhaps he didn't think it was necessary. Old-school thinking was that you couldn't infect someone else when the virus was dormant and you didn't have blisters. Not true! We now know that once you are infected, you risk transmitting the virus to a partner every time you have sex. Of course, even being fully warned wouldn't have entirely protected my patient had she still had sex, but at least she wouldn't have been blindsided by an infection.

I suspect many of us could have made this same mistake or misjudgment. She was afraid of offending, but now who is offended? She was afraid of appearing distrustful, but do you think she will ever blindly trust another partner again? I am not sure what ended up happening to their relationship, but I imagine that this episode led to the hasty conclusion of a love story that otherwise might have had a chance. See my rules for Smart Sex earlier in this chapter so nothing like this ever happens to you!

HUMAN IMMUNODEFICIENCY VIRUS (HIV)

Back in the 1980s when acquired immunodeficiency syndrome (AIDS) was first detected in this country and traced to infections by the Human Immunodeficiency Virus (HIV), it was virtually a death sentence. It also almost exclusively affected homosexual males. In the decades since then, there have been tremendous advances in treatment options that allow infected people to live well for many years without succumbing to AIDS, which is the most advanced stage of an HIV infection, or contracting any of the so-called "opportunistic infections" such as meningitis, tuberculosis, and a type of cancer called Karposi's Sarcoma that prey on a person when the immune system is compromised.

Another change, however, is that heterosexual as well as homosexual men and women are now being infected with HIV. Children born of infected mothers are at risk as well. Also, a recent study by the

Centers for Disease Control and Prevention (CDC) showed that the annual HIV infection rate is 40 percent higher than was previously estimated. You need to know about this viral STI just as much as you need to know about the ones we've already discussed. A 2008 report from the American College of Physicians (ACP) notes that 20 percent of infected Americans are over age fifty and 20 percent have partners who didn't know they had an infection. As a result, the ACP recommends that almost everyone over the age of thirteen be screened for HIV. That means all of us!

Causes of HIV

HIV is contracted through sexual contact, blood, and body fluids including breast milk. Partners who share needles may get HIV from blood. Years ago people got HIV from blood transfusions but now blood banking is so sophisticated that infected blood is identified and thrown out.

Symptoms of HIV

According to the Centers for Disease Control and Prevention, the following may be indicators of the presence of an HIV infection:

- rapid weight loss
- dry cough
- recurring fever or profuse night sweats
- profound and unexplained fatigue
- swollen lymph glands in the armpits, groin, or neck
- diarrhea that lasts for more than a week
- white spots or unusual blemishes on the tongue, in the mouth, or in the throat
- pneumonia
- red, brown, pink, or purplish blotches on or under the skin or inside the mouth, nose, or eyelids
- memory loss, depression, and other neurological disorders

Diagnosis of HIV

There is an FDA-approved kit called the Home Access Express HIV-1 Test System that you can use by yourself. The FDA recommends this home test and reports that the results have been shown to be highly accurate. You prick your finger and let the blood dry on a special paper and then send the sample in the included mailer to a laboratory for analysis. You include the anonymous personal identification number (PIN) that came with your kit. In a few weeks you get the results by telephone using your PIN. Free counseling is included in the telephone call after you learn the results. The kit is available at brick-and-mortar and online drugstores for $40 to $60.

The FDA warns that all other home tests for HIV are unapproved. Claims of a visual sign of your results such as a red dot appearing within five to fifteen minutes are entirely bogus.

If you prefer, you can have your own doctor give you an HIV test or you can visit the CDC's Web site (cdc.gov) to find testing centers near you. The home test only checks for antibodies, and your immune system takes up to eight weeks to develop them after exposure to HIV. If you want results sooner than that, there is a test that your doctor can order that detects elements of the actual HIV virus. This sensitive test can turn positive within a few days after infection. (See "How Not to Get STIs," earlier in this chapter, for information about having a potential new partner tested for HIV.)

Treatment of HIV

There are currently a number of drug "cocktails" consisting of several medications that are proving in combination to be quite effective in controlling HIV. The most widely used combination is the "highly active antiretroviral therapy" (HAART). This treatment uses three anti-retroviral drugs (ARVs). Most often, two of the three are nucleoside or nucleotide reverse transcriptase inhibitors (NRITs) and the third one is either a non-nucleoside reverse transcriptase inhibitor (NNRTI) or a protease inhibitor (PI).

If you managed to read all of the above, congratulations! I'm pretty sure you don't need anything any more detailed than that mouthful of medical terms to convince you that help is at hand if you have HIV. Suffice it to say that there are individual therapies tailored to the specific needs of each patient. As always, be as detailed as possible when you report your symptoms to your doctor and ask every question that comes to mind (or that you were wise enough to write down before your visit) so that you can get the best care possible.

Also, remember that HAART and any of the other regimens available are not cures. All they do is keep the HIV infection at bay. If you take them intermittently or stop them because you're feeling better, the infection will recur.

BACTERIAL INFECTIONS

Bacterial STIs can by and large be cured with antibiotics. However, they are often "silent" or asymptomatic. Testing is essential for anyone at risk. Left untreated, bacterial STIs can lead to conditions that can cause chronic problems and infertility.

CHLAMYDIA

Chlamydia is the most common sexually transmitted infection. Any sexually active person can be infected with the chlamydia bacteria, although young girls and young women are at much higher risk than older women. This is because chlamydia likes to infect the mucous-producing tall columnar lining cells of the transformation zone. In younger females, the zone extends out of the cervix and is thus more easily exposed to chlamydia during sex. In older women, the zone is usually found inside the donut hole. (See diagram on page 11.)

Seventy to 90 percent of women and over half of men who have chlamydia will develop no symptoms at all. That doesn't mean there isn't trouble brewing under the surface. There often is. For this reason, chlamydia is called a "silent" disease. If symptoms do occur, they usually appear within one to three weeks after exposure to the bacteria.

Symptoms of Chlamydia

The bacteria can infect the cervix (cervicitis) and the urethra (urethritis). Cervicitis frequently causes no symptoms. Even if the infection spreads from the cervix to the fallopian tubes, there may still be no symptoms. However, you may experience the following:

- abnormal vaginal discharge
- burning during urination
- lower abdominal pain
- low back pain
- nausea
- fever
- pain during intercourse
- bleeding between menstrual periods

Chlamydia infection of the cervix can also spread to the rectum even without anal sex.

If chlamydia is not treated, an infection can progress to serious problems such as infection of the uterus or fallopian tubes causing pelvic inflammatory disease (PID). (For information about the diagnosis and treatment of PID, see chapter 7.) Postmenopausal women with low estrogen rarely get PID because their cervical opening is often narrow and tightly closed ("stenotic") due to atrophic estrogen-depleted cells. PID can cause permanent damage to the fallopian tubes and uterus and can lead to chronic pelvic pain, infertility, and a tubal or ectopic pregnancy (see chapter 5). Infection of the fallopian tubes with chlamydia causing subsequent scarring and blockage is one of the main causes of infertility.

Women are frequently reinfected if their partners are not treated. Men are less likely than women to be checked for chlamydia, as men aren't programmed to go to their doctors for an annual checkup the way women are.

All sexually active women age twenty-five years and younger should be tested yearly for chlamydia. This is a strong guideline. It is so important that doctors are rated according to whether they follow this rule or not. An annual screening test is also recommended for women over twenty-five who have a new partner or partners. If you fall into that category, at your next gynecology visit let your doctor know you want to have a test for chlamydia.

Diagnosing Chlamydia

There are a number of urethral or cervix swab and urine tests that are reliable for identifying a chlamydia infection. For many years, doctors relied on cultures to test for chlamydia, but cultures require specialized handling and laboratory procedures. Today there are many tests that detect the presence of chlamydia through antigen or DNA testing without doing a culture. Urine tests allow for routine checks for chlamydia without a pelvic examination or swab test, but this is a much less reliable way to discover hidden chlamydia in both women and men.

Treatment of Chlamydia

Chlamydia can easily be treated and cured with antibiotics. A single dose of azithromycin or a week of doxycycline twice daily are the most commonly used treatments.

What works:

- Azithromycin (Zithromax) 1 g orally in a single dose
- Doxycycline 100 mg orally twice a day for seven days
- Erythromycin 500 mg orally four times a day for seven days
- Erythromycin 800 mg orally four times a day for seven days
- Floxin (ofloxacin) 300 mg orally twice a day for seven days
- Levaquin (levofloxacin) 500 mg orally once daily for seven days

Your partner should be evaluated, tested, and treated. If you have chlamydia, you should abstain from sexual intercourse until you and your partner have finished treatment.

GONOCOCCAL INFECTIONS (GONORRHEA, OR GC)

Gonorrhea is the second most common bacterial STI. Women ages twenty-five and younger are at highest risk for GC but older women with new partners should also get tested. GC infections in women frequently cause no symptoms until serious complications, including pelvic inflammatory disease (PID), occur (see chapter 7).

The majority of infections in men result in a thick puslike discharge and pain of the urethra that causes them to seek treatment soon enough to prevent problems. Unfortunately, that's often not soon enough to protect their partners from getting infected because the symptoms may not occur for up to thirty days after a GC infection is acquired.

Symptoms of GC

Women who do experience symptoms of a vaginal GC infection may believe that they have a urinary tract infection (UTI or cystitis) since the symptoms can be similar (see chapter 9). GC can also infect the anus and bowels and the throat. The latter infection causes virtually no symptoms but can be passed on to a partner through oral sex. For vaginal and rectal (anal) GC, the symptoms may be:

- burning sensation during urination
- yellowish vaginal discharge
- discharge or bleeding from the anus

Diagnosis of GC

A swab of cervical or vaginal discharge, if there is any, is sent to a laboratory for testing. This is not a routine test like the one for chlamydia, so if you believe you are at risk, at any age, ask for the test!

Treatment of GC

GC infections of the cervix, urethra, and rectum respond well to the following antibiotics:

- Ceftriaxone (Rocephin) 125 mg shot in a single dose
- Cefixime (Suprax) 400 mg orally in a single dose
- Ciprofloxacin (Cipro) 500 mg orally in a single dose
- Ofloxacin (Floxacin) 400 mg orally in a single dose
- Levofloxacin (Levaquin) 250 mg orally in a single dose

SYPHILIS

Syphilis is a relatively uncommon but curable sexually transmitted infection caused by a type of spirochete bacteria called *Treponema pallidum*. Like the other bacterial STIs, syphilis is often asymptomatic. Most cases of syphilis are effectively treated with antibiotics.

Symptoms of Syphilis

Legend has it that the origin of the modern necktie is the high ruffled collar fashionable in Shakespeare's time, which was purportedly worn to cover the telltale red rash of syphilis that was dubbed the "Collar of Venus." Whether that is so or not, here is the earliest symptom that may occur:

- a chancre sore or sores on the genitals and/or anus

This is the primary phase and it will go away on its own, but unless you get treatment, syphilis will progress to the secondary phase, which includes:

- a reddish brown rash that doesn't itch and may appear in various places on the body including the neck, the hands, and the soles of the feet
- fever
- swollen lymph glands
- sore throat

- bald patches
- headaches
- unexplained weight loss
- aching muscles
- unexplained fatigue

Left untreated, syphilis will go into a latent phase with no symptoms. This phase can last ten or fifteen years. After that, however, syphilis kicks in again, potentially causing serious damage to internal organs as well as blindness, dementia, and even death.

Diagnosis of Syphilis

In the primary stage, your doctor can use a microscope to examine material taken from a chancre sore if one is visible. This procedure allows your doctor to identify the characteristic bacteria. A more reliable diagnosis, and the only one for asymptomatic syphilis, is an inexpensive blood test that shows the presence of antibodies to the syphilis bacteria.

Treatment of Syphilis

In the early stages, penicillin is the most effective treatment. If you are allergic to penicillin, your doctor may suggest skin testing or referral to an infectious-disease expert to see if penicillin would be safe. It is far and away the best treatment for syphilis.

TRICHOMONIASIS ("TRICH")

Trich is grouped with the bacterial STIs but it is actually not caused by a bacterium but rather by the protozoan *T. vaginalis*, a single-celled organism with flagella. These are long, thin appendages that the organism uses to propel itself. Under a microscope, *T. vaginalis* can be seen swimming around in a smear of vaginal discharge. The organism is larger and more complex than a bacterium. Fortunately, as with bacterial STIs, trich can be cured with antibiotics.

In contrast to chlamydia and GC, which are most often seen in young women, trichomoniasis is common in women of all ages. A study of trich in Denmark showed the average age of women reported to have trichomoniasis to be thirty-nine years old, compared with twenty-four years and twenty-two years for women with GC and chlamydia, respectively. However, like GC and chlamydia, trich is often asymptomatic.

Symptoms of Trichomoniasis

Although not all women with trich will have symptoms, the most common symptoms include:

- heavy, yellow-green vaginal discharge
- irritation of the vulva

Diagnosis of Trichomoniasis

There are over-the-counter tests that you can use to check whether your vagina or vaginal discharge has an abnormally high pH count. (See chapter 7 for information about other conditions that can cause a high pH count.) If your pH is high, see your doctor. Be aware, however, that blood—including menstrual blood—and semen can raise the pH temporarily, so don't use the tests during your period or after sex. And please, if the test is normal but you still have symptoms, see your doctor anyway.

In addition to a general medical history and pelvic exam, your doctor will examine any vaginal discharge under a microscope to look for the very familiar protozoa swimming about. Unfortunately this method has a sensitivity of only 60 to 70 percent. There are new FDA-approved tests for trichomoniasis in women that doctors can use as well. Although these tests tend to be more sensitive than looking under the microscope, false positives occasionally occur.

In the final analysis, a culture is the best method of diagnosis. For women in whom trichomoniasis is suspected but not confirmed by the microscope exam or other tests, any vaginal discharge should be cultured for *T. vaginalis*.

Treatment of Trichomoniasis

The oral nitroimidazoles (metronidazole/Flagyl and tinidazole/Tindamax) are the only class of drugs used for treatment of trichomoniasis. They result in cure rates of approximately 90 to 100 percent. Treatment of your partner is necessary to guarantee this success rate, however. I usually write a prescription for my patient and her partner although it is always good advice to have your partner check in with his doctor or pharmacist to assure that there are no contraindications to treatment.

Here are the antibiotics that work:

- Metronidazole (Flagyl) in a single 2 g dose orally or 500 mg orally twice a day for seven days
- Tinidazole (Tindamax) as a single 2 g oral dose

The good news is that trich is easy to treat but only if you strictly adhere to three straightforward but not always easy to follow rules:

- Don't have sex while being treated.
- Have your partner treated as well.

Women Who Have Sex with Female Partners

There is very little research on the risk of STIs as a result of sex between women, but the risk probably depends on the specific infection and the sexual practice. For example, a shared penetrative item such as a vibrator may be a possible means for transmission of infected vaginal discharge.

Transmission of HPV can occur with skin-to-skin or skin-to-mucosa contact, which can happen during sex between women. Also, many women who have sex with other women have also had sex with men and therefore should undergo all the usual STI precautions and testing, including the Pap test.

- Do not consume alcohol during treatment and until twenty-four hours after completion of metronidazole therapy or seventy-two hours after completion of tinidazole therapy.

Metronidazole gel, a topical treatment, is considerably less effective for the treatment of trichomoniasis with cure rates under 50 percent. Topically applied medication probably does not get into the urethra or perivaginal glands and so is not very effective.

You probably noticed that throughout this chapter I recommended that you should talk with your doctor about all the issues involved in Sex Smarts, including STIs. Still, don't think I'm not aware that this is easier said than done. Not only are patients uneasy when it comes to having frank discussions about their sexual history and complaints, but many doctors are squeamish as well. Dr. Margaret Blythe, head of the American Academy of Pediatrics Committee on Adolescence, remarked during a briefing after the news broke about the alarming prevalence of STIs among teen girls that "some doctors mistakenly think, 'Sexually transmitted diseases don't happen to the kinds of patients I see.'"

Sadly, this attitude is not the exclusive province of doctors who treat girls and young women. Any doctor may have similar blinders on. A recent study reported in the *New England Journal of Medicine* showed that only one in five women felt able to discuss sex with her doctor. Yet as you have read in this chapter, much can be learned about solutions and treatments for everything from reduced libido to STIs by having conversations with your doctor. For that matter, talking with your doctor in a way that commands respect for you and your questions and opinions is vital to successful outcomes for all of the problems we'll be addressing in the later chapters of this book.

Let's move on, then, to the very important next chapter, "How to Get the Health Care You Need at Every Age."

3

How to Get the Health Care You Need at Every Age

IN THIS CHAPTER

- Talking with Your Doctor

- Collecting Copies of Your Medical Records

- Having Gynecologic Exams

- Going for Your Annual Physical

- What Does "Blood Work" Mean?

- What Is a Mammogram?

- Should I Have Genetic Testing?

- What Is a Bone Density Test?

No one is in a better position than you are to make sure you get the best health care possible. First of all, no one cares more about your health than you do. Second, although your doctor and your other health-care providers are well-trained experts in their medical disciplines, you are the one and only expert about how you feel and whether or not the way you feel is different enough from normal to send up a red flag. Third, you are the one who knows the full details of your lifestyle, your family history, and your health history. Finally, you are legally entitled to copies of your medical records—everything from your blood work to your bone density X-rays to your hospital discharge papers. If you don't collect and organize as complete a set of those records as possible, no one will.

But don't worry. Getting your records isn't all that difficult and learning to communicate your "health story" to your doctor isn't very hard either. I'm here to give you the confidence and know-how you need in order to help your health-care providers help you.

TALKING WITH YOUR DOCTOR

If you're typically a little intimidated in the presence of your doctor, you're not alone. There is even a documented phenomenon called the "White Coat Syndrome" in which a patient's blood pressure spikes dramatically when she's tested in a physician's office even though her blood pressure is normal when she measures it herself at home. The age-old notion of the doctor on a pedestal still exists for many women, even those who are empowered "squeaky wheels" in other aspects of their lives such as relationships, careers, and finances. Also, most of us are anxious about submitting to examinations that require getting naked and wrapping ourselves in robes left open in front. We're also worried that we might learn some bad news. Then there's the issue of stepping on a scale in front of someone who's going to write down how much you weigh. And that's just the office visit! If you end up needing to go to a hospital, your anxiety level is pretty much guaranteed to escalate even more. No wonder people have trouble relaxing enough to open up to their doctors. Still, you can't get the care you need unless you give your doctor detailed information and ask questions. The key is to arrive for your visit well prepared. Here's how:

WRITE YOUR HEALTH HISTORY AND BRING IT WITH YOU
When you show up for an appointment at a medical facility, you'll probably be handed a pen and a clipboard with forms to fill out even if you've been there before. If you're admitted to a hospital, you'll have a stream of interns, residents, "hospitalists" who specialize in hospital medicine, nurses, and doctors all coming into your room and asking

the same questions over and over about your health history. I recommend bringing along print-outs of your health history that you have typed and saved on your computer ahead of time. Getting all the facts down in advance is a great way to make sure you don't miss anything. You can copy the information onto whatever forms you're required to fill out by hand. You can also refer to your typed list when you need to answer questions. I have forms posted on my Web site (www.drsavard .com) that you can download and fill out for free. However, you can simply type the following information in a format that works for you. Be sure to update your documents periodically when details such as dates and dosages of medications change.

Basic Information

List your full name, maiden name if applicable, gender, date of birth, relationship status, and contact information for yourself and an emergency contact.

Insurance

List your carrier and your policy number.

Current Medical Conditions

If you have any known problems, even if they are well controlled with medication and/or lifestyle choices, list them here. Examples are diabetes, hypertension (high blood pressure), high cholesterol, osteoporosis, and a heart murmur that requires antibiotics with dental work.

Previous Illnesses

Go back as far as you can remember including childhood illnesses such as measles and mumps if you grew up before the vaccines for those conditions were available. If you've ever had pneumonia, put that on the list. Also, be sure to include STIs (see chapter 2, page 38).

Surgeries

Include non-invasive techniques, arthroscopy, and major surgery. (A cesarean section is major surgery even if you had a "bikini" incision.")

Menstrual and Reproductive History

List the following:

- the date of your first period (menarche)
- details about your cycles such as how many days typically elapse between periods, whether your flow is light or heavy, whether you have painful cramps, and whether you experience PMS that affects your quality of life
- dates of pregnancies, if any, including miscarriages and any problems such as preeclampsia or gestational diabetes
- information about your childbirth experiences, if any, such as a vaginal deliveries, C-sections, induced labor, forceps, preterm labor, precipitate labor, inefficient labor
- gender of your children, whether they are twins or other multiples, and whether any babies were stillborn
- dates of abortions, if any
- if you are currently trying to get pregnant, the date that you started
- information about assisted reproductive technology (ART) if you have tried or are trying to get pregnant this way or if you have given donor eggs
- if you are currently pregnant, the date that you're due
- method of contraception if you are trying not to get pregnant
- methods of contraception previously used
- conditions, past or present, such as fibroids, pelvic inflammatory disease (PID), and endometriosis
- signs of perimenopause, if any, such as mood swings and irregular, heavy periods, hot flashes, night sweats, and vaginal dryness
- the date of your final period if you have gone through menopause

Hospitalizations

List the admitting and discharge dates for all your hospitalizations as well as the reasons for your hospital stays or out-patient (ambulatory) procedures.

Immunizations

- Tetanus and diphtheria. You need a shot every ten years so keep track of when you had your last one.
- Diptheria/Pertussis/Tetanus (DPT). You need one once as an adult as a booster because Pertussis (whooping cough) is on the rise. This combination shot is in addition to the tetanus and diphtheria shots you need every ten years.
- Flu. Vaccinations for new influenza strains are available once a year and they're recommended for all adults over age fifty and anyone with a chronic disease, and for health-care workers and caregivers living with or caring for people with chronic illnesses. However, I think just about everyone would be wise to get the shot.

Is It Okay to Get Immunizations at "Retail Clinics"?

Chain stores such as Wal-Mart and some drugstores have clinics staffed by nurses, nurse practitioners, and occasionally by doctors. A study done at the University of Pennsylvania School of Medicine found that most people who visit the clinics don't have primary care practitioners (PCP) or family doctors. I hope you do have a PCP, but if not, you can safely get your shots at one of these "retail clinics." You can also have your blood pressure checked and get routine lab tests such as blood work and urinalysis. The other reasons patients typically go to the clinics, according to the study, are for colds, bronchitis, earaches, conjunctivitis (pink eye), and urinary tract infections (cystitis).

- Pneumonia. For people over sixty-five, there is now a vaccination available. You only need to get it once, or a booster if you received an earlier pneumonia vaccine years ago.
- HPV vaccination: a series of three shots over six months. (See chapter 2.)
- Shingles vaccine. A vaccine that reduces the risk of the painful and dreaded complication of the chickenpox virus in about half of those who are inoculated is now available. The vaccine is for adults age sixty and over. You only need to get it once.
- Meningitis vaccine. You need it once usually during adolescence or before going off to a college dorm, where you are most likely to be exposed to the deadly bacteria.
- You can also list childhood and special travel vaccinations if you can remember them or have a record of them. Examples are hepatitis A and B, typhoid, chicken pox, and measles.

Tests

See "Going for Your Annual Physical" later in this chapter for the tests you need depending on your age. List the dates and results of your most recent tests, if any, for the following:

- Pap test (see chapter 2)
- HPV test (see chapter 2)
- mammogram
- bone density test
- colonoscopy
- blood work
- urinalysis
- EKG
- blood pressure
- stress test
- CT scan to check for calcium build-up or plaque in the heart arteries

Name							Date of Birth	
DATE								Target Goal
Height/Weight								
BMI (Body Mass Index)								
Waist Circumference								
Blood Pressure								
Blood Glucose								
Total Cholesterol								
HDL (good)								
LDL (bad)								
Triglycerides								
TSH (Thyroid)								
Rectal Exam								
Stool for Blood								
Sigmoid/Colonoscopy								
Breast Exam								
Mammogram								
Pap Test								
HPV with Pap								
Total Skin Exam								
Vision Exam								
Dental Exam								
Bone Density Exam (Osteoporosis)								
Change in Medication or Treatment								

Other tests to discuss with your doctor: Complete blood count, urinalysis, EKG and hearing test.

Test Results at-a-Glance Form

Allergies

List and describe any known allergies or reactions to the following:

- medications
- food, especially nuts and seafood
- bee stings
- dyes used in medical tests
- pet dander
- pollen
- dust

Medications and Supplements

List everything you take whether prescription or over-the-counter, including vitamins and herbal supplements. Include dosages and directions. Make one list for what you take daily and another for what you take occasionally.

Substance Use

Create an honest report about the frequency and amount of your use of the following substances. The written list is for your eyes only, but sharing the information with your doctor can be important:

- tobacco
- recreational drugs
- alcohol

Your doctor can tell you about the health effects of "pack years" if you currently smoke or have quit smoking cigarettes and she can also tell you about "joint years" if you currently smoke or have quit smoking marijuana. If your alcohol consumption is higher than recommended (no more than a drink a day for women) or if you are a binge drinker, she can tell you what your health risks are.

Weight Gain or Maintenance

Your weight as well as the circumference of your waist ("belly fat") are important factors in the "health story" you share with your doctor. Indicate whether or not you have experienced unexplained weight loss. Also note whether or not you watch your weight successfully or have not been able to control your weight. The ideal waist circumference for women is around thirty-one inches or at least under thirty-five inches (see chapter 11). (For men, the ideal is less than thirty-seven inches or at least under forty inches). Waist size is considered the new vital sign along with temperature, pulse, and blood pressure. You can also find your body mass index (BMI) using calculators on the Internet such as the one at the Centers for Disease Control Web site, http://tinyurl.com/b53foz.

A BMI between nineteen and twenty-five is optimal and over thirty is obese.

Exercise Regimen

Indicate whether you lead a sedentary, moderately active, or very active lifestyle and list your types of physical activity.

Sex

List whether you are sexually active, whether or not you are in a committed relationship or have multiple partners, and whether you have male or female partners. Remember, you don't have to hand this list to anyone so don't be afraid to write down the information. Sharing it with your doctor during a conversation with her can be important. Studies have shown that if you don't tell, your doctor won't ask.

Family Medical History

Family history matters most if your relatives had early onset or premature incidences of diseases such as diabetes, heart disease, strokes,

Which Health Information Should I Carry with Me?

Just about everyone carries a health insurance card, but few people carry the information that could save their lives in an emergency. Make a list of the following items and keep it with you at all times. Also, post a copy on your refrigerator. That's where EMS workers are trained to look when they respond to 911 calls.

- medical conditions such as hypertension, diabetes, osteoporosis, even a heart murmur that requires antibiotics before dental work
- serious adverse reactions to medication, bee stings, seafood, nuts, and X-ray dye
- an up-to-date list of medications, vitamins, and herbal supplements, including dose and directions
- significant family medical conditions
- blood type if you know it
- most recent immunizations for tetanus, flu, and pneumonia
- living-will information
- emergency contact
- a copy of your most recent EKG

or cancer. For example, if your mother developed heart disease before the age of sixty-five or your father had it before the age of fifty-five, you are at a greater risk than normal because heart disease "runs in the family." However, if your mother died because her heart stopped at the age of ninety, you're not at a higher than normal risk for cardiac arrest. Everybody's heart stops eventually. This is why, insofar as you can recall or find out, you need to list not only your relatives' serious illnesses and causes of death but also their ages at death. Include, if possible, your parents, your paternal grandparents, your maternal grandparents, your aunts and uncles on both sides of the family, and your siblings.

Also, don't forget that alcoholism is a disease. If you are prone to it because of your family history, you may be more likely to become addicted to other substances, too. Your doctor can avoid prescribing potentially addictive medications for you.

Advance Directive

If you have an advance directive or "living will," note where it is kept and who has your Durable Power of Attorney for Health Care.

Health-Care Providers Contact List

Include your primary care physician, your gynecologist, your dentist, your optometrist or ophthalmologist, and any specialists and complementary care clinicians such as mental-health-care providers, physical therapists, orthopedic surgeons, cardiologists, urologists, acupuncturists, and chiropractors.

KEEP A HEALTH JOURNAL

When I give speeches or talk with my own patients, I often use the following quote from Albert Schweitzer, M.D., the noted physician who was also a philosopher, musician, and theologian:

> Each patient carries his own doctor inside him. They come to us not knowing that truth. We are at our best when we give the doctor who resides within each patient a chance to work.

You can help your doctor do exactly that if you trust your instincts and pay attention to what I call your "health radar." Keep track of your symptoms, hunches, and concerns in a health journal that you can print out and share with your doctor. Simply jot down notes and date them. Examples might be:

- "I saw some blood in my stool. I think I have a hemorrhoid. I always seem to get them when I'm on my feet a lot. I went to a string of holiday parties last week where I was standing up for hours so that's probably the reason."
- "My last period was eight days late. I was freaking out about starting my new job so I think that's why."
- "I've been taking a blood pressure med for several years but I never had any side effects until yesterday. My feet swelled so much that I couldn't get my shoes on. Maybe I need a lower dose? Or maybe it was just the heat? I was visiting family in Arizona."
- "I noticed a fishy odor coming from my vagina starting last week. Bathing doesn't help."
- "I haven't been feeling like myself lately. Nothing specific, but I just feel kind of low and not motivated."

KEEP A HEALTH CALENDAR

Enter the dates you're due for everything from an annual Pap test to a new tetanus shot to your first mammogram or bone density test. Your doctor may be keeping track of these dates as well, but maybe not. In any case, if you move or you switch doctors because you get a new insurance plan at a new job, or you step on a nail and end up in the emergency room when you're away from home on a summer vacation, you'll be all set to ask for the shots and tests you need. (See "Going for Your Annual Physical" later in this chapter for a list of shots and tests for each decade of your life.)

MAKE A LIST OF SYMPTOMS AND QUESTIONS

For every office visit, arm yourself with a written list of anything that's bothering you. Consult your health journal and also use the symptoms lists in chapters 7, 8, and 9 as guides for ways to describe what you're experiencing. I know that talking about "female problems" can be embarrassing, but a good doctor is comfortable examining and discussing what's "down there." Also, if you're hesitant to describe symptoms that could be caused by an STI or an unhealthy lifestyle change, remember that your doctor isn't there to judge you. She's there to make a diagnosis and to use her medical knowledge and skill to help you. So speak up!

For every office visit, arm yourself with a written list of anything that's bothering you.

Also, don't be afraid to ask questions if you've done some research and you want clarification about what you've found. Studies done by iCrossing and Burst Media showed that almost 80 percent of women turn to the Web when they have a health issue. That's wonderful in the sense that more and more women are being proactive about their health, but the Internet is not always a reliable source of information. If you run across worrisome data or community message boards with scary stories, tell your doctor about your concerns. He'll be able to sort the bogus information from the truth. Also, medicine is a fast-paced field and you just might have run across legitimate breaking news that your doctor hasn't yet seen. If so, he'll welcome the chance to investigate further and possibly find more current treatment options for you. And if he doesn't react that way, consider going to a different doctor. The long-standing paradigm of the all-knowing physician as the authority figure doesn't work anymore. No doctor these days should roll his eyes when a patient wants to be a partner in her own care.

WRITE DOWN WHAT YOUR DOCTOR TELLS YOU

A study reported in the *Journal of General Internal Medicine* showed that most patients forget 50 percent of what a doctor has said as soon as the appointment is over. Don't let that happen to you. Take notes during your office visit and enter them in your health journal and health calendar once you get home. Of course, taking notes isn't always easy during an examination or when you're rattled by a scary diagnosis. See my next tip about asking someone to come with you.

BRING ALONG A "HEALTH BUDDY"

Even the most powerful, assertive person can be afraid of what she'll hear from the doctor or simply forget to ask or speak up. That's why you would do well to enlist the help of someone you trust to be your "health buddy." Most of us have a girlfriend, daughter, sister, or mother who's perfect for this role. You can return the favor when she needs to see her doctor or have a test she's dreading. There's nothing like the supportive presence of someone you love to bolster your courage and make sure you give and get all the information you need. Incidentally, I have found in my practice that women seldom bring their husbands as health buddies but that men do bring their wives. My gynecologist friends, however, say that husbands come along for pregnancy- and fertility-related visits.

Your health buddy can take over the job of checking off the items on the lists you bring with you and she can be the one who takes notes. That frees you to relax as much as possible without worrying that you're missing something. She can also make sure your doctor knows that you want to receive copies of your test results and she can hand him your stamped, self-addressed envelope. The next section of this chapter explains why this is so important.

COLLECTING COPIES
OF YOUR MEDICAL RECORDS

Take the following quiz:

True ☐ False ☐   If your doctor doesn't let you know the results of tests, that means "no news is good news" so there's no need to make a follow-up phone call.

True ☐ False ☐   Your test results and medical records are on file all together somewhere in a computer.

True ☐   False ☐   Test results are almost never misplaced, misread, or misfiled.

True ☐   False ☐   Doctors you saw previously always send your complete records to your new doctor or to a hospital.

True ☐   False ☐   Doctors and pharmacists will always warn you about potentially harmful interactions among your prescribed medication and certain other prescription and over-the counter drugs including herbal remedies.

If you answered "True" to any or all of the above, you're in for a shock. You—not your doctor, pharmacist, or hospital—are the only one responsible for the accuracy and completeness of your medical records. I have long preached this message. In 2008 two papers from the University of Chicago that were published in the June issue of *Quality and Safety in Health Care* confirmed my assertions. A study of eight family practice clinics found an "unacceptable" level of mistakes in ordering, implementing, and reporting medical tests.

Not only that, but doctors and many institutions are only required to keep your records for as short a time as seven years before destroying them. Yet 80 percent of the diagnoses your doctor makes comes from the history he has in front of him. Imagine the difficulty of making a diagnosis, let alone recommending the right treatment, if information is unavailable, incorrect, or incomplete. As a family doctor I found out firsthand the importance of my patients taking an active role in their health care and keeping copies of their health information. Many of my patients had complex problems requiring multiple doctors. Some of them were spending winters in the Sunbelt, which meant they saw a different doctor for half the year. A lot of them were seeing complementary care practitioners and using complementary therapies. However, new patients often came for an initial office visit with no paperwork at all. I had no concrete data to go on—no consultation reports from doctors, no X-ray reports, no test results, no list of medications or immunizations, no history of allergic reactions, no hospital discharge summaries.

One Woman's Story: Judy, Age 42

"I had a gyn exam and a Pap smear every January without fail from the time I was in my first relationship when I was twenty-two. I never called my doctor for the test results because I figured he'd let me know if anything was wrong. Then last year when I went for my annual exam, my doctor came in with my chart and started reading it. All of sudden he was frowning. He looked up and said, 'Judy, you had an abnormal Pap test last year. Didn't you get our letter?'

"I was horrified! I said, 'What letter? I never got one!' The doctor scheduled me for a test called a colposcopy so he could do a biopsy. I was a wreck back home while I was waiting for the lab results. I would look at my wonderful husband and my two girls, who were nine and twelve at the time, and just burst into tears. I couldn't bear the thought of having cancer and leaving them behind. If only I had asked for a copy of my results a year earlier and read them myself! As it turned out, I did have cervical cancer but I was lucky in the sense that the cancer had not yet spread beyond the pelvic area. I had a hysterectomy and I'm fine.

"Fortunately my family was complete. But believe me, I will never again assume that no news is good news when it comes to test results. Now I always give my doctor a stamped self-addressed envelope so I can get copies of my results. I do the same for my husband and kids. What a simple way to stay on top of our most important asset—our own health!"

When I first launched my campaign to get patients to collect and organize their own medical records, most people were surprised to learn that they are legally entitled to copies of those records. Since then, the 2003 federal Privacy Rule, added to the 1996 Health Insurance Portability and Accountability Act (HIPAA) of 1996, has made clear that you can, as the government site puts it, "ask to see and get a copy of your health records" and "have corrections added to your health records." The law also gives you the right to control how providers and insurers share your information for various purposes. However, you can now only get records for yourself and your minor children. Anyone else in your charge, such as an aging parent or an adult child still living with you, needs to sign a document that designates you as someone with the right to his or her health information.

Despite the fact that you are legally entitled to copies of your records, you may be afraid that you'll antagonize your doctors and hospital personnel by requesting copies. Rest assured, however, that when I speak to most doctors on this topic, they react with enthusiasm and relief. They understand immediately that patients who collect and study their own records and who make it their business to become well informed about their health concerns will be in a better position to join forces with them instead of worshipping them or seeing them as the enemy.

Incidentally, studying your records is an important aspect of this process. You may think you won't be able to understand them, but for the most part they are written in plain English. Any terms you don't understand can be researched on the Internet or in a medical dictionary. Also, throughout this book you'll find actual examples of test results so you'll be familiar with them when you get your own. Believe me, the time and effort you take to go over your records will be well worth it. Some people discover incorrect information about medications and allergies. Others learn that their doctors overlooked critical findings in the results of X-rays or blood tests. Still others discover misleading information in their records or notice that important information is missing.

LOCATING YOUR MEDICAL RECORDS

As I said earlier, your records may have been destroyed if seven or more years have elapsed since you had the tests. Don't panic. Try to find your past records, but if they're not available, you can simply start now and keep collecting records as you go along.

Be sure to give your date of birth when you request your records since that's how they're filed. I suggest that you offer $10 to cover administrative time and copying costs and always include a stamped self-addressed envelope. The records to look for and where to get them are described below.

Your Family Doctor and Your Gynecologist

Ask for the following:

- Progress notes, including a running record of your height, weight, and blood pressure (Doctors who still make handwritten notes may not want to give you copies because their writing is pretty much illegible. However, many doctors now type their notes on computers or dictate them and have them transcribed. Whatever the case, I'd politely insist on getting copies of the notes.)
- Summaries dictated by specialists you've seen, such as cardiologists, gynecologists, or urologists
- Discharge summaries from hospital stays and emergency room treatment
- Results of blood work and urinalysis

Do I Need to List My Blood Type?

List it if you know it but don't be concerned if you don't. Should you ever need a transfusion, medical personnel will do a test to verify your blood type.

EXERCISE STRESS TEST

INDICATION:

  Atypical chest pain

PROCEDURE:

  The patient exercised for 8 minutes and 30 seconds on the Bruce protocol, stopping due to fatigue and arrhythmias. Chest pain did not occur .

FINDINGS:

  Resting heart rate was 61 and blood pressure 112/72. Physical examination was normal.

  At peak exercise the heart rate was 160 (90% of age predicted maximum) and the blood pressure was 145/70 mmHg.

  Functional capacity is normal. The normal range for 62 year old men is 6'50 - 10'15 on the Bruce protocol.

  Resting ECG revealed normal findings .

  During exercise ST segment changes did not occur.

  There were no arrhythmias .

CONCLUSIONS:

  1. Negative ECG test for ischemia .
  2. Chest pain did not occur .
  3. Arrhythmias did not occur .
  4. Nuclear agent was not injected .
  5. Normal functional capacity.

Cardiac stress test results

- Pathology (laboratory) reports such as Pap tests and biopsies
- Radiologists' reports, such as chest X-rays, mammograms, and bone density scans. You may also want to get a copy of the actual X-ray pictures along with the typed reports. This is especially important for women who move and need to have mammograms read and compared at another facility.
- Results of heart testing: EKG and cardiac stress test
- Results of screening and diagnostic tests such as allergy testing and colonoscopy

- Immunization history. If your doctor doesn't have this, blood tests can determine which antibodies you have as a result of some but not all vaccines.

Specialists

If your family doctor has not received consultation reports from your specialists, you'll need to contact the specialists directly. Also, if you see a specialist regularly, such as a cardiologist, make a habit of getting your results on an ongoing basis just as you do when you visit your family doctor or gynecologist.

Dear ____ ,

Thank you for referring your patient for evaluation of her dyslipidemia.

As you know she is a 21-year-old white female college student with a benign past medical history. She has never smoked, drinks socially and although she's active gets minimal significant aerobic exercise. In the past, she has had an unrestricted diet and does have a predilection for lipid rich foods.

In the spring of 1993 she saw an ophthalmologist for routine exam and a "plaque" was seen and she was advised to have a lipid profile. In May, 1993 her total cholesterol was 324, triglycerides 247, HDL 50, LDL 225, ratio 6.4 and her apo-B was 228. She saw a nutritionist and modified her diet and when she saw you in August, 1993 her lipids had improved somewhat. You noted that she was also taking birth control pills and I believe you instructed her to stop them. Secondary causes of dyslipidemia were ruled out with normal thyroid function, liver function test and sugar. Her last lipids before seeing me showed continued improvement with her cholesterol down to 258 but with her HDL also dropping as is sometimes noted with dieting.

Her family history does show the death of her grandfather at the age of 67 from MI and the death of her paternal uncle at the age of 38 from a stroke. Her other uncle age 48 is alive and well with normal lipids. Her father has mild hypercholesterolemia but no coronary heart disease. Her mother age 45 is also free of disease and has normal lipids. Her grandfather reportedly has dyslipidemia and is currently being treated with Mevacor although her grandmother and aunt are alive and well without dyslipidemia.

Her other medical problems include mild hypercalcemia which is asymptomatic and a PTH was normal.

Example of a specialist's consultation report

Hospital Medical Records Departments

In the event that your family doctor doesn't have your hospital discharge summaries, contact the medical records department at the hospital and specifically request *only the summary*. Otherwise, you may get (and be charged for) the whole file, which will be redundant.

THOMAS JEFFERSON UNIVERSITY HOSPITAL

Attending Physician: ▓▓▓▓▓▓▓▓▓▓▓▓

DISCHARGE SUMMARY

FINAL DIAGNOSIS: Methicillin-sensitive staphylococcus aureus, buttock abscess.

HISTORY AND PHYSICAL: CHIEF COMPLAINT: Left buttock abscess.

HISTORY OF PRESENT ILLNESS: A 55-year-old female with a history of hepatitis C, chronic pancreatitis, migraines, osteoarthritis, and irritable
bowel syndrome, presented with a 9-day history of a left buttock erythematous lesion, which was painful and had been increasing in size; originally the size of a quarter, no covering most of her buttock area. She did have associated fevers to 102.7 and chills, no history of trauma,
no skin breakdown; also a history of recurrent pustular lesions in that area since 01/2007, which were previously treated with Keflex.

ALLERGIES: GADOLINIUM CAUSES A RASH.

MEDICATIONS: Topamax 50 mg p.o. b.i.d.; Viactiv 2 tablets p.o. daily; Nexium 40 mg p.o. b.i.d.; Fioricet 2 tabs p.o. p.r.n.; Fosamax; Percocet 1-2 tabs q.4-6 hours p.r.n.; Valium 5 mg p.o. at bedtime p.r.n.; Allegra 180 mg p.o. daily; Prilosec 40 mg p.o. at bedtime; Prempro daily; and a zinc supplement daily.

PAST MEDICAL HISTORY: Hepatitis C, chronic pancreatitis, migraines, osteoarthritis, and irritable bowel syndrome - diarrhea type.

PAST SURGICAL HISTORY: C-section, tonsillectomy, shoulder repair.

SOCIAL HISTORY: Alcohol socially, no tobacco, no IV drug use.
Occupation:
Medical secretary.

Example of a hospital discharge summary

Laboratory or Hospital Radiology Departments

If your family doctor doesn't have your laboratory results or X-rays, you can try contacting the lab or hospital radiology department.

Complementary Care Clinicians

Contact all of the complementary care clinicians you see, including nutritionists, acupuncturists, physical therapists, and chiropractors.

Now you know how to prepare for office visits, what to bring along, and what to ask for when you're there. If you're healthy and not pregnant, you may only need your annual visit to your gynecologist starting when you become sexually active and a periodic visit to your family doctor for a physical. Here's what to expect during those visits.

Should I Store My Medical Records Online?

There are several options available on the Internet for storing your medical records. One of the more highly touted services promises links so that you can get your records electronically from doctors, hospitals, and pharmacies. However, very few links are in fact offered. In addition, do you really want your most private information stored on a Web site, no matter how secure it purports to be? Even more important, hard copies of your records, organized in a loose-leaf binder or file folders, can be handed to anyone from a new doctor to an emergency responder to your daughter acting as Durable Power of Attorney. No one has to boot up a computer or fiddle with a USB drive. With all due respect to President Obama's vision of having electronic health records for everyone in the United States within five years, I predict that privacy issues and cost will continue to stall that initiative for the foreseeable future. Hard copies are still your best bet.

HAVING GYNECOLOGIC EXAMS

Most women schedule an annual gynecologic exam. Unless you're a teenager who hasn't yet had a "pelvic," you know what happens but you may not know the reasons for this important checkup. Here's a reminder of what you'll experience, plus information about what your doctor is looking for during each part of the exam:

- You undress and wrap yourself in a gown that you leave open in front.
- Then you lie on your back on the examining table, put your feet in the stirrups, and open your legs.
- The doctor shines a light and inserts an instrument called a speculum into your vagina so that she can expand it and see inside. She is looking for changes in the shape and size of your vagina and cervix. (See chapter 1 for descriptions of these organs.) She's also looking for signs of STIs (see chapter 2) and other infections.
- She will collect a sample of cells from your cervix for a Pap smear and for an HPV test if needed (see chapter 2). The procedure doesn't hurt, but the speculum is usually cold and you may feel a little tug or cramp when the doctor takes the cell sample.
- After she removes the speculum, she'll do a "bimanual" or two-handed exam by inserting two gloved fingers of one hand into your vagina and placing her other hand on your abdomen. She'll "palpate," meaning press and feel, in search of any growth or areas that cause you pain.
- Next she'll insert a gloved finger into your rectum to check for abnormalities. She'll ask you to roll over on your side for the rectal exam if not you're not already up in stirrups.
- She'll also perform a breast exam as part of the appointment. Be sure you do monthly self-exams of your breasts as well. A study

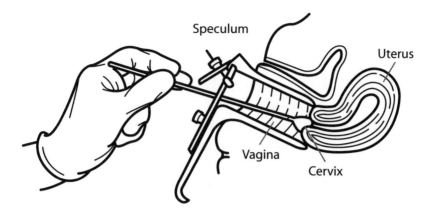

Pelvic exam with speculum

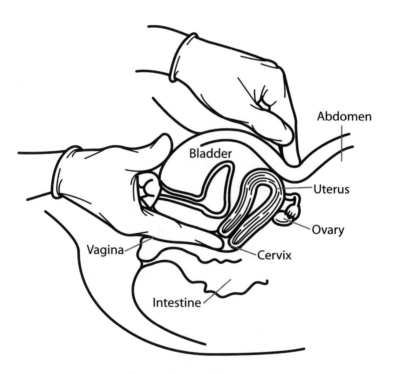

Bimanual gynecologic exam

that got a lot of attention by claiming that women shouldn't examine their own breasts was almost universally denounced by the medical community and women alike. True, self exams may occasionally cause a woman to go for a biopsy because she finds a lump that turns out to be benign. However, many women detect cancerous lumps at the earliest stages and are therefore able to be treated successfully for this most feared and common of female cancers.

GOING FOR YOUR ANNUAL PHYSICAL

A lot of women think that a yearly gynecological exam is sufficient preventive care. However, I firmly believe that you need a periodic physical with a primary care physician (PCP)—a family doctor or an internal medicine physician like me who is trained to treat you holistically. She will screen you for cardiovascular risk, bone density, cancer risks, emotional and psychological issues, weight issues, lifestyle habits, and immunizations.

Here are the tests and examinations you should have at each decade of your life in addition to your gynecologic exam, which should include your Pap test if you are sexually active as well as a rectal exam and a breast exam (see above).

STARTING IN YOUR TWEENS AND TEENS

- A checkup every two or three years.
- DPT (diphtheria/pertussis/tetanus) booster
- HPV vaccine, best before your "sexual debut." This is approved for girls as young as nine. (See chapter 2.)
- Meningitis vaccine. This is required by many colleges for incoming freshmen.

STARTING IN YOUR TWENTIES

- Annual Pap test starting three years after you first become sexually active or by age twenty-one
- A "head-to-toe" physical every three to five years

  1. Examination of the skin over your entire body to check for signs of skin cancer
  2. Blood pressure check
  3. Height, weight, and waist circumference
  4. Blood work (See What Does "Blood Work" Mean?, page 105.)
  5. Mental Health Assessment
  6. Cardiovascular Risk Assessment, meaning your family history; your personal habits such as smoking, activity, and diet habits; lipids; blood sugar; and waist size.

- Dental exam. The exams, which you've probably been getting every six months since childhood, check for decay and plaque buildup and look for signs of inflammation and infection. Chronic periodontal disease increases the risk of several diseases including heart disease and tonsillar cancer from an HPV infection. Regular flossing between dental checkups is important.
- Vision. This exam checks for vision and any treatable retina or other eye problems.

STARTING IN YOUR THIRTIES

In addition to the list you started in your twenties, have a test for the presence of HPV at the same time you have your Pap test. The same swab of material from the cervical transformation zone used for your Pap test can be put in liquid and tested for the high-risk strains of HPV. (Don't confuse this test with the vaccine for HPV. Even if you got the HPV vaccine, you still need a regular Pap test and/or an HPV test to check for cervical cancer because the vaccine does not protect against all cancer-causing strains. See chapter 2, page 44.)

STARTING IN YOUR FORTIES

Add an annual mammogram.

STARTING IN YOUR FIFTIES

Add the following:

- Colonoscopy. This examination of the colon with a flexible, lighted tube should be performed every ten years to help screen for colon cancer. You may also opt for a so-called "virtual colonoscopy," an X-ray that is not invasive and that is much less expensive than the traditional procedure. Recent research has shown that the virtual colonoscopy is now almost as effective as a regular colonoscopy, at least when the X-ray procedure is performed by top experts in the field. Virtual colonoscopy, however, is more likely to miss the often cancerous flat-type tumors that are much more difficult to spot on an X-ray and are reported to be on the rise.

- Stool occult blood test. This test is designed to find hidden (occult) blood in your stool. You do it yourself at home using stool cards and sending them to a laboratory. Your doctor will give you the cards with instructions. The presence of blood can signal precancerous or cancerous polyps in the colon, or intestinal bleeding from such causes as a stomach ulcer, internal hemorrhoids, or severe colitis. Women age fifty or older should do this test every year. If you have a family history of polyps, colon cancer, or severe colitis, you can begin doing the test at age forty or five years earlier than the age of disease onset for any family member.

- EKG. A baseline electrocardiogram (EKG) to assess your heart's electrical activity should be done by age fifty. This serves as a reference to be compared with future EKGs that will be done if you have symptoms. You should carry a copy of your baseline

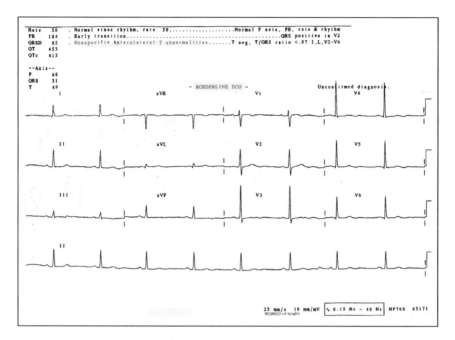

A Normal Electrocardiogram (EKG)

EKG along with your health information (see "Collecting Copies of Your Medical Records" earlier in this chapter.)

- If you are at increased risk for heart disease because of your family history, ask for an ultrafast CT scan to check the calcium score of your arteries. You may also ask for a stress test, which checks the electrical activity of your heart with exercise. Unfortunately a stress test is often not reliable, especially in women. Some women who have severe heart disease will have a perfectly normal stress test.

STARTING IN YOUR SIXTIES

Add the following:

- Bone density test. Women age sixty-five or older (or those fifty or older who are at increased risk because of family history) should have a bone density test to screen for osteoporosis.

- Blood test for vitamin D level. Most older women will have low results, and this can jeopardize their bones, brains, and hearts as well as increase the risk of autoimmune diseases and cancers. It is easily treated with vitamin D supplements, however.

WHAT DOES "BLOOD WORK" MEAN?

Your blood contains a great deal of information about your health. When your doctor orders the lab to run a complete series of tests, you can find out about the status of your liver, your thyroid, your blood cholesterol, your blood sugar, and much more. An overnight fasting sample is best so your doctor will schedule you for first thing in the morning and tell you not to eat breakfast.

COMPLETE BLOOD COUNT (CBC)

This is the most common blood test but it's actually optional. Your doctor may order it as part of a complete physical examination. He'll also order it before you have surgery and if you have unexplained and continuing symptoms. The complete blood count (CBC) measures the number, size, and shape of the different types of cells in your blood and checks for anemia (low red blood cells) and inflammation/infection (high white blood cells).

BLOOD CHEMISTRY TESTS

A single sample of your blood serum can be used to run a series of tests quickly and inexpensively. The following explains the most commonly requested tests:

- Glucose can indicate diabetes if your level is high or hypoglycemia if it's low. A fasting glucose of less than 100 is normal, a level of 100 to 125 is abnormal and called "impaired glucose tolerance" or prediabetes, and a level of 126 or greater means diabetes.

- Blood urea nitrogen and creatinine are tests of your kidney function.
- Sodium, potassium, and chloride are blood salts or electrolytes. These tests are especially important if you are on diuretics ("water pills") for hypertension or heart disease.
- Uric acid is a waste product of all cells. An elevated level may mean kidney disease or gout.
- Albumin is a blood protein produced by your liver. A low albumin count can be a sign of liver or kidney disease.
- Globulin is a blood protein produced by your immune system. A high count can point to chronic inflammation, infection, or blood disorders such as multiple myeloma.
- Calcium is a component of your blood that helps all the cells in your body function normally. Your blood calcium level has nothing to do with how much calcium is in your bones. A high count can point to a disorder called hyperparathyroidism, which predisposes you to kidney stones and low bone density.
- Serum glutamine pyruvic transaminase (SGPT) and serum flutamate oxaloacetate transaminase (SGOT) are enzymes (proteins) produced primarily by the liver. SGOT is also produced by red blood cells.
- Lactate dehydrogenase (LDH) is an enzyme produced by many cells of the body. If this test result is extremely high, your doctor will want to do additional tests, depending on your specific complaints, to rule out a malignancy.
- Bilirubin is the chemical in bile that gives it its yellow color. If the bile passages from the liver to the intestine are blocked, your bilirubin level will be high. Possible causes include gallstones and liver disease.
- Gamma glutamyl transpeptidase (GGT) is an enzyme produced by the liver. Obesity and excessive alcohol use are the most common reasons it can be mildly increased. It will

also be elevated when there is blockage of bile and with liver disease.

- Alkaline phosphatase is an enzyme produced by the liver and bones. If it is abnormal (elevated), looking at the GGT (see above) will help determine the source. If the GGT is elevated as well, the liver is the culprit. People with fatty liver from excess visceral fat may first be alert to it when routine blood tests show elevated liver enzymes (assuming you don't drink in excess, a common cause of liver disease).
- C-reactive Protein (CRP). Women at increased risk for metabolic syndrome and heart disease (women with waist circumference over 35 inches) should ask for the high-sensitivity C-reactive protein test—an important test of blood inflammation and marker of future heart disease risk. A CRP under 1.0 is low risk.
- Blood Fats. Also called lipids, these are often listed together in a separate "panel" on your blood chemistry report. Sometimes only the total cholesterol and perhaps the triglyceride level will be listed if your doctor didn't specifically request results for the lipid panel. However, you need all your numbers in order to make the best evaluation for heart disease.
- Total cholesterol is the sum of your LDL and HDL (see below). High total cholesterol levels are linked to heart disease. The lower your total cholesterol, the better. A total below 200 is desirable. However, some women have such a high level of "good cholesterol" that the total is over 200. In these cases, the number is a not a warning sign.

> **High-density lipoprotein (HDL)** is your "good cholesterol." Remember, "high density should be high." The more of this type, the better. Ideally, your HDL cholesterol should be at least 30 percent of your total

amount. In men, an HDL greater than 40 is normal; in women, an HDL greater than 50 is normal.

Low-density lipoprotein (LDL) is your "bad choles- terol." Remember, "low density should be low". A high LDL puts you at risk for heart disease; your doctor will suggest diet and sometimes medication to get your LDL cholesterol below 130. If you have diabetes or heart dis- ease already, your treatment goal for LDL cholesterol should be below 100. Some research suggests that if you have diabetes, severe heart disease risk, or recent heart attack, you should target an LDL of under 70.

Triglycerides are the other form of fat in your blood. The level will be much higher after a meal. If your level is out of range, it should be repeated after an overnight fast. Ele- vated levels both fasting and even after a meal increase your risk of heart disease and could be a sign of early diabetes. Ideally they should be under 150. Postprandial (after a meal) elevated triglycerides are now thought to be especially worrisome for women whereas years ago we used to say they were okay even if elevated.

- Thyroid function tests include three measures: the levels of two hormones produced by the thyroid glands—thyroxine 3 (T3) and thyroxine 4 (T4), and the thyroid stimulating hormone (TSH) level. T3 and T4 regulate your metabolism. The brain keeps levels normal by sending TSH to the thyroid gland if your T3 and T4 are low. The TSH level is the best indicator of the condition of your thyroid and the effects of thyroid medication. For example, if your thyroid hormone levels (T3 and T4) are low, the TSH level will be high. If the thyroid hormone levels are too high, then the TSH level will be low or immeasurable.

Test Name	Results	Units	Reference Range	Site
30163E TSH - Thyroid	3.9	MU/L	0.4- 4.2	

83A COMP METABOLIC PANEL

	Results	Units	Reference Range	Site
CALCIUM	8.9	MG/DL	8.4- 10.2	
GLUCOSE — "sugar"	104	MG/DL	65- 109	
UREA NITROGEN	12	MG/DL	7- 23	
CREATININE "kidney"	0.8	MG/DL	0.6- 1.5	
BUN/CREATININE RATIO	15		7- 24	
PROTEIN,TOTAL	7.3	G/DL	6.0- 8.2	
ALBUMIN	4.2	G/DL	3.5- 5.0	
GLOBULIN,CALCULATED	3.1	G/DL	1.9- 3.8	
A/G RATIO "liver"	1.4		0.9- 2.1	
BILIRUBIN,TOTAL	0.3	MG/DL	0.2- 1.4	
ALKALINE PHOSPHATASE	88	U/L	25- 125	
AST	20	U/L	1- 40	
SODIUM "electrolytes"	135	MEQ/L	134- 145	
POTASSIUM		MEQ/L	3.5- 5.3	

Specimen was received uncentrifuged or incompletely centrifuged. The
resulting prolonged contact with cells may adversly affect some
components of a chemistry screen
POTASSIUM VALUE ABOVE 5.0 MEQ/L. FALSE ELEVATION MAY OCCUR IF SERUM IS
NOT SEPARATED FROM CLOT WITHIN 1 HOUR OF VENIPUNCTURE.

	Results	Units	Reference Range	Site
CHLORIDE	95	MEQ/L	96- 107	
CARBON DIOXIDE	30	MEQ/L	21- 31	

968T LIPID PANEL - Blood Fats

	Results	Units	Reference Range	Site
CHOLESTEROL,TOTAL	252	MG/DL	120- 199	
TRIGLYCERIDES	214	MG/DL	40- 199	
HDL CHOLESTEROL	47	MG/DL	35- 60	
CHOLESTEROL/HDL RATIO	5.4		2.40- 5.35	
LDL CHOLESTEROL,CALC	162	MG/DL	75- 130	

Comprehensive Blood Test results

19131189
CENTER FOR WOMENS HEALTH,
MONROE OFFICE CTR-STE 100
ITY LINE & PRESIDENTIAL WAY
HILA PA 19131-

Laboratory Report

SB **SmithKline Beecham**
Clinical Laboratories

Patient Name	Patient ID/Hospital ID	Room No.	Age	Sex	Physician
			45	F	SAVARD, MARIE
	Ref No.	Collection Date & Time	Log-in Date		Report Date & Time
		11/02/94 9AM	11/02/94		11/11/94 18:00
Remarks					

Report Status	Test	Result In Range	Out of Range	Units	Reference Range	Site Code
FINAL						
	CUSTOM PROFILE 305					
	CHEMZYME PLUS					KP
	GLUCOSE		58 L	MG/DL	70-115	
	SPECIMEN SLIGHTLY HEMOLYZED.					
	UREA NITROGEN (BUN)	9		MG/DL	7-25	
	CREATININE	0.8		MG/DL	0.7-1.4	
	BUN/CREATININE RATIO	11.3		(CALC)	6.0-25.0	
	SODIUM	139		MEQ/L	135-146	
	POTASSIUM	4.7		MEQ/L	3.5-5.3	
	CHLORIDE	104		MEQ/L	95-108	
	MAGNESIUM	2.0		MEQ/L	1.2-2.0	
	CALCIUM	10.1		MG/DL	8.5-10.3	
	PHOSPHORUS, INORGANIC		5.3 H	MG/DL	2.5-4.5	
	PROTEIN, TOTAL	7.5		GM/DL	6.0-8.5	
	ALBUMIN	4.4		GM/DL	3.2-5.0	
	GLOBULIN	3.1		GM/DL (CALC)	2.2-4.2	
	A/G RATIO	1.4		(CALC)	0.8-2.0	
	BILIRUBIN, TOTAL	0.5		MG/DL	0-1.3	
	ALKALINE PHOSPHATASE	34		U/L	20-125	
	LACTATE DEHYDROGENASE	210		U/L	0-250	
	GGTP	4		U/L	0-45	
	CONFIRMED IN DUPLICATE					
	AST (SGOT)	29		U/L	0-42	
	ALT (SGPT)	15		U/L	0-48	
	URIC ACID		2.4 L	MG/DL	2.5-7.5	
	IRON, TOTAL	132		MCG/DL	25-170	
	IRON BINDING CAPACITY	308		MCG/DL (CALC)	200-450	
	% SATURATION	42.9		% (CALC)	12.0-57.0	
	SOME OF THE ABOVE RESULTS MAY HAVE BEEN					
	AFFECTED BY THE PRESENCE OF RED BLOOD					
	CELLS IN THE SERUM.					
	TRIGLYCERIDES	77		MG/DL	<200	
	CHOLESTEROL, TOTAL	182		MG/DL	<200	
	HDL-CHOLESTEROL					KP
	HDL-CHOLESTEROL	67		MG/DL	>OR=35	
	SPECIMEN SLIGHTLY HEMOLYZED.					

(Continued)

Page 1 of Complete Blood Work

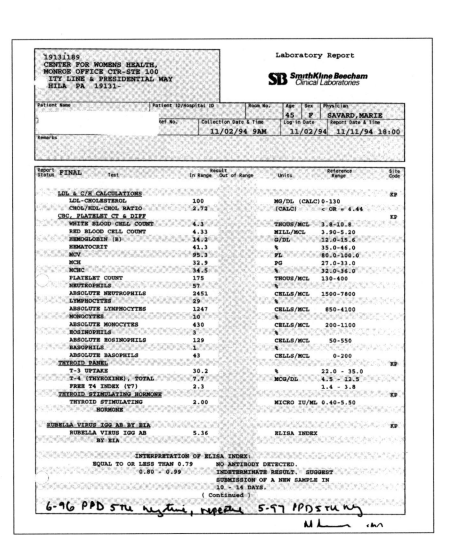

19131189
CENTER FOR WOMENS HEALTH,
MONROE OFFICE CTR-STE 100
ITY LINE & PRESIDENTIAL WAY
HILA PA 19131-

Laboratory Report

SB SmithKline Beecham
Clinical Laboratories

Patient Name	Patient ID/Hospital ID		Room No.	Age	Sex	Physician
				45	F	SAVARD,MARIE
	Ref No.	Collection Date & Time		Log-in Date	Report Date & Time	
		11/02/94 9AM		11/02/94	11/11/94 18:00	

Remarks

Report Status FINAL	Test	Result In Range	Out of Range	Units	Reference Range	Site Code
LDL & C/H CALCULATIONS						KP
	LDL-CHOLESTEROL	100		MG/DL (CALC)	0-130	
	CHOL/HDL-CHOL RATIO	2.72		(CALC)	< OR = 4.44	
CBC, PLATELET CT & DIFF						KP
	WHITE BLOOD CELL COUNT	4.3		THOUS/MCL	3.8-10.8	
	RED BLOOD CELL COUNT	4.33		MILL/MCL	3.90-5.20	
	HEMOGLOBIN (B)	14.2		G/DL	12.0-15.6	
	HEMATOCRIT	41.3		%	35.0-46.0	
	MCV	95.3		FL	80.0-100.0	
	MCH	32.9		PG	27.0-33.0	
	MCHC	34.5		%	32.0-36.0	
	PLATELET COUNT	175		THOUS/MCL	130-400	
	NEUTROPHILS	57		%		
	ABSOLUTE NEUTROPHILS	2451		CELLS/MCL	1500-7800	
	LYMPHOCYTES	29		%		
	ABSOLUTE LYMPHOCYTES	1247		CELLS/MCL	850-4100	
	MONOCYTES	10		%		
	ABSOLUTE MONOCYTES	430		CELLS/MCL	200-1100	
	EOSINOPHILS	3		%		
	ABSOLUTE EOSINOPHILS	129		CELLS/MCL	50-550	
	BASOPHILS	1		%		
	ABSOLUTE BASOPHILS	43		CELLS/MCL	0-200	
THYROID PANEL						KP
	T-3 UPTAKE	30.2		%	22.0 - 35.0	
	T-4 (THYROXINE), TOTAL	7.7		MCG/DL	4.5 - 12.5	
	FREE T4 INDEX (T7)	2.3			1.4 - 3.8	
THYROID STIMULATING HORMONE						KP
	THYROID STIMULATING HORMONE	2.00		MICRO IU/ML	0.40-5.50	
RUBELLA VIRUS IGG AB BY EIA						KP
	RUBELLA VIRUS IGG AB BY EIA	5.36		ELISA INDEX		

INTERPRETATION OF ELISA INDEX:
EQUAL TO OR LESS THAN 0.79   NO ANTIBODY DETECTED.
0.80 - 0.99   INDETERMINATE RESULT. SUGGEST
SUBMISSION OF A NEW SAMPLE IN
10 - 14 DAYS.
(Continued)

6-96 PPD 5TU negative, repeated 5-97 1PDS TU neg

Page 2 of Complete Blood Work

19131189
CENTER FOR WOMENS HEALTH,
MONROE OFFICE CTR-STE 100
CITY LINE & PRESIDENTIAL WAY
HILA PA 19131-

Laboratory Report

SB **SmithKline Beecham**
Clinical Laboratories

Patient Name	Patient ID/Hospital ID	Room No.	Age	Sex	Physician
			45	F	SAVARD,MARIE
	Ref No.	Collection Date & Time	Log-in Date	Report Date & Time
Remarks		11/02/94 9AM	11/02/94	11/11/94 18:00

Report Status	FINAL	Test	Result In Range Out of Range	Units	Reference Range	Site Code

```
                      1.00 - 2.89         LOW LEVEL OF ANTIBODY DETECTED.
                      2.90 - 6.59         MODERATE LEVEL OF ANTIBODY DETECTED
          EQUAL TO OR GREATER THAN 6.60   HIGH LEVEL OF ANTIBODY DETECTED.

      THE PRESENCE OF ANTIBODY SUGGESTS PREVIOUS INFECTION OR VACCINATION
      WITH RUBELLA VIRUS.

      IF RECENT INFECTION IS SUSPECTED, THE TEST FOR RUBELLA IGM ANTIBODY
      IS RECOMMENDED.

      IN ADDITION, ANTIBODY LEVELS IN ACUTE AND CONVALESCENT PHASE (PAIRED)
      SERA MAY BE TESTED CONCURRENTLY TO DETERMINE IF THERE HAS BEEN A
      RECENT OR CURRENT RUBELLA INFECTION.
```

HEPATITIS B SURFACE ANTIBODY (QL)   KP
      HEPATITIS B SURFACE   POSITIVE   NONE DETECTED
          ANTIBODY (QL

                              CONFIRMED IN DUPLICATE

HEPATITIS A AB, TOTAL   KP
      HEPATITIS A AB, TOTAL   NONE DETECTED
                          NONE DETECTED

VARICELLA ZOSTER, ELISA   KP
      VARICELLA ZOSTER, ELISA   0.39

                  EXPLANATION OF ELISA VALUES
            0.12 OR LESS   NO ANTIBODY DETECTED--
                                SUGGESTS ABSENCE OF PRIOR
                                EXPOSURE TO VZ
            0.13 TO 0.14   EQUIVOCAL RESULT--
                                TO OBTAIN A DEFINITIVE
                                RESULT WE SUGGEST A NEW
                                SERUM SPECIMEN BE
                                SUBMITTED FOR TESTING
            0.15 TO 0.28   LOW LEVEL OF ANTIBODY
                                    (Continued)

Page 3 of Complete Blood Work

Laboratory Report

SB SmithKline Beecham
Clinical Laboratories

19131189
CENTER FOR WOMENS HEALTH,
MONROE OFFICE CTR-STE 100
CITY LINE & PRESIDENTIAL WAY
HILA PA 19131-

Patient Name	Patient ID/Hospital ID	Room No.	Age	Sex	Physician
			45	F	SAVARD,MARIE

	Ref No.	Collection Date & Time	Log-in Date	Report Date & Time
		11/02/94 9AM	11/02/94	11/11/94 18:00

Remarks

Report Status FINAL	Test	Result In Range	Out of Range	Units	Reference Range	Site Code
			DETECTED			
	0.29 TO 0.53		MODERATE LEVEL OF ANTIBODY			
			DETECTED			
	0.54 OR GREATER		HIGH LEVEL OF ANTIBODY DETECTED			

ELISA VALUES OF 0.15 OR GREATER SUGGEST PRIOR EXPOSURE TO
VARICELLA ZOSTER. PATIENTS WITH ACTIVE VARICELLA INFECTION
MAY NOT SEROCONVERT FOR UP TO 4 DAYS AFTER ONSET OF VESICLES.
TEST DETECTS IGG CLASS OF ANTIBODIES.

RUBEOLA VIRUS IGG AB BY EIA   KP
    RUBEOLA VIRUS IGG AB   0.61
        BY EIA

            EXPLANATION OF ELISA VALUES
        0.13 OR LESS   NO ANTIBODY DETECTED--
                              SUGGESTS ABSENCE OF PRIOR
                              EXPOSURE TO MEASLES
        0.14 TO 0.15   EQUIVOCAL RESULT--
                              TO OBTAIN A DEFINITIVE RESULT
                              WE SUGGEST A NEW SERUM
                              SPECIMEN BE SUBMITTED
                              FOR TESTING
        0.16 TO 0.29   LOW LEVEL OF ANTIBODY
                              DETECTED
        0.30 TO 0.52   MODERATE LEVEL OF ANTIBODY
                              DETECTED
        0.53 OR GREATER   HIGH LEVEL OF ANTIBODY DETECTED

ELISA VALUES OF 0.16 OR GREATER SUGGEST PRIOR EXPOSURE TO
OR VACCINATION AGAINST MEASLES. PATIENTS WITH ACTIVE
MEASLES INFECTION MAY NOT SEROCONVERT FOR UP TO 4 DAYS AFTER
ONSET OF RASH. TEST DETECTS IGG CLASS OF ANTIBODY.

(Continued)

Page 4 of Complete Blood Work

WHAT IS A MAMMOGRAM?

A mammogram is an X-ray that can detect breast cancer early, often before a lump can be felt. Some women find the exam painful. A new study reports that the application of a topical anesthetic, Lidocaine, can be helpful. Schedule this test the week after your period when your breasts will be least tender and glandular. If you are taking hormone therapy after menopause your breasts may appear more glandular or dense from the hormones. Ask your doctor about stopping the hormones a few weeks before the scheduled test.

Women between the ages of forty and forty-nine should have this test every one or two years and women over fifty should have it yearly. Women at high risk for breast cancer because of family history and women with dense breasts should ask about a digital mammogram and for some women, an MRI. More facilities than ever have a digital mammogram machine, so ask for it in advance of appointment.

SHOULD I HAVE GENETIC TESTING?

If you have a strong family history of a disease, you may want to have DNA tests done to see whether you were born with genes that predispose you to that disease. However, be wary of companies that offer genetic testing but are not regulated by state health departments. If you do want testing, ask your doctor for a referral to a legitimate medical facility.

- For hereditary breast and ovarian cancer, the BRCA 1 and 2 tests are helpful but only predict less than 5 percent of all cancers. Many women who test positive now opt to help prevent cancer by having prophylactic surgery to remove ovaries and/or breasts (double mastectomies/oophorectomies).
- There is a test available for Alzheimer's disease but it does not

Bryn Mawr Hospital
Main Line Health

COMPREHENSIVE BREAST CENTER

Founders Building
101 S Bryn Mawr Ave
Bryn Mawr, PA 19010
(610) 526-4400

Patient Name
Date of Birth:
X-Ray Number:
Date of Exam: 07/27/2005
Accession Number: 4074115   Order Number: 90003
Attending Physician: BRADLEY W FENTON   Status: O
Ordering Physician: BRADLEY W FENTON   Room/Bed: -

Final Report

ACR CODE:

CLINICAL HISTORY: Screening.

PROCEDURE: OBD 0202 - 07/27/2005 - SCREEN MAM DIRECT DIGITAL BILAT   76083

COMMENT: Comparison is made with the previous digital examination of 2004. Full field digital mammography with computer assisted detection was performed. When compared with the prior study, no suspicious change is seen. The patient does have older studies at home which would allow extended comparison and this is suggested. The patient was asked in writing to submit the previous studies for more extended comparison in a routine manner. There are scattered benign appearing calcifications bilaterally. There is nodular tissue within the upper aspect of the right breast which is unchanged.

IMPRESSION:
Nothing suspicious seen on today's examination.
The patient will be supplying earlier studies for more extended comparison.

FINAL ASSESSMENT BIRADS CATEGORY 0 - INCOMPLETE: NEEDS ADDITIONAL COMPARISON WITH OUTSIDE STUDIES (OSFN DG)

Mammography reports should be evaluated with the following in mind:
1. A report that is negative for malignancy should not delay biopsy, if there is a dominant or clinically suspicious mass. Some cancers are not visualized by mammography.
2. In dense breasts, an underlying mass may be obscured.
3. Ultimate diagnosis of malignancy is histologic.

D: Jul 27 2005 4:14P T: Jul 28 2005 8:20A DPC

Trans By: DPC: Jul 28 2005 8:20A
Dictated By: JOHN STASSI M.D.: Jul 27 2005 4:14P
Dictation signed by: JOHN STASSI M.D.: Jul 28 2005 8:50A

Report Receivers:
BRADLEY W FENTON - (030114)
FRANCES R BATZER - (030979)

Diagnostic Imaging	Harry G. Zegel, MD		BATCH :
Appts: (610) 526-4500	Chairman, Main Line Health Imaging Services		Process: Jul 28 2005 8:50AM
Nuc Med (610) 526-3530	Emma Simpson, MD	Harry G. Zegel, MD	Robert Pinsk, MD
File Room (610) 526-8737	Director, Bryn Mawr Hospital	Director, Lankenau Hospital	Director, Paoli Hospital

Mammogram report

detect the risk for all patients and there is no specific treatment to prevent the disease.

- If you have Huntington's disease in your family, you have probably already been counseled about the pros and cons of testing and have made a deeply personal decision.

WHAT IS A BONE DENSITY TEST?

This is an X-ray, also called the DXA scan, which measures your bone density. The lower your bone density, the greater your risk for bone fractures. (There is also a much less accurate heel ultrasound test that does *not* diagnose osteoporosis but merely tells your doctor whether you are at risk and should have the more complete DXA scan test.)

The DXA scan is considered the gold standard for the diagnosis of osteoporosis. The most important score or result to check is your T-score. The T-score tells you how your bones compare to that of a

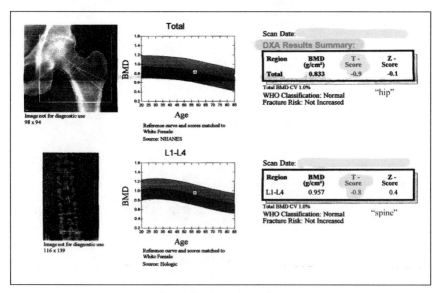

Bone density test results

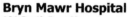

Bryn Mawr Hospital
101 South Bryn Mawr Avenue
Bryn Mawr, PA. 19010

Patient:	Patient ID:	
Birth Date:	Physician:	
Height / Weight:	Measured:	:05 PM (8.80)
Sex / Ethnic:	Analyzed:	:13 PM (8.80)

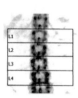

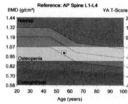

Region	BMD (g/cm²)	Young-Adult (%)	T-Score	Age-Matched (%)	Z-Score
L1	0.771	68	-3.0	75	-2.1
L2	0.931	77	-2.3	84	-1.4
L3	1.048	86	-1.4	95	-0.5
L4	1.134	93	-0.7	102	0.2
L1-L4	0.987	83	-1.7	91	-0.8

Image not for diagnosis

Matched for Age, Weight (females 25-100 kg), Ethnic
NHANES (ages 20-30) / USA (ages 20-40) AP Spine Reference Population (v102)
Statistically 68% of repeat scans fall within 1SD (± 0.010 g/cm² for AP Spine L1-L4)

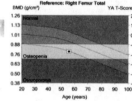

Region	BMD (g/cm²)	Young-Adult (%)	T-Score	Age-Matched (%)	Z-Score
Neck	0.714	69	-2.3	80	-1.3
Troch	0.661	78	-1.7	87	-0.9
Shaft	0.917	-	-	-	-
Total	0.785	78	-1.8	85	-1.1

Image not for diagnosis

Matched for Age, Weight (females 25-100 kg), Ethnic
NHANES (ages 20-30) / USA (ages 20-40) Femur Reference Population (v102)
Statistically 68% of repeat scans fall within 1SD (± 0.012 g/cm² for Right Femur Total)

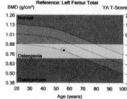

Region	BMD (g/cm²)	Young-Adult (%)	T-Score	Age-Matched (%)	Z-Score
Neck	0.708	68	-2.4	79	-1.3
Troch	0.674	79	-1.5	89	-0.8
Shaft	0.936	-	-	-	-
Total	0.797	79	-1.7	87	-1.0

mage not for diagnosis

Matched for Age, Weight (females 25-100 kg), Ethnic
NHANES (ages 20-30) / USA (ages 20-40) Femur Reference Population (v102)
Statistically 68% of repeat scans fall within 1SD (± 0.012 g/cm² for Left Femur Total)

GE Medical Systems
LUNAR

Prodigy
DF+16078

DXA scan of the spine and hip, test results

Bryn Mawr Hospital
Main Line Health

DIAGNOSTIC RADIOLOGY REPORT

Outpatient Imaging
101 S Bryn Mawr Ave
Bryn Mawr, PA 19010
(610) 526-8700

Patient Name:
Date of Birth:
X-Ray Number:
Date of Exam: 07/27/2005
Accession Number: 4073762
Attending Physician: BRADLEY W FENTON
Ordering Physician: BRADLEY W FENTON

Order Number: 90002
Status: O
Room/Bed: -

Final Report

ACR CODE:

CLINICAL HISTORY: Post menopausal. 627.2.

PROCEDURE: OXR 6075 - 07/27/2005 - DEXA BONE DENSITY STUDY

Scans of the lumbar spine and both hips were obtained. The bone mineral density was calculated for all the levels scanned. The patient's bone mineral density was referenced to both young normal patients (T-score) as well as age matched patients (Z-score). For the evaluation of osteoporosis, it is recommended that the patient's bone mineral density be compared to young normal patients or the T-score.

Current World Health Organization criteria for the diagnosis of osteoporosis is as follows:
1. Up to 1 standard deviation below normal compared to young normal patients - normal.
2. Between 1 and 2.5 standard deviations below normal compared to young normal patients - low bone mass or osteopenia.
3. Greater than or equal to 2.5 standard deviations below normal compared to young normal patients - osteoporosis.

COMMENT: Scanning of the lumbar spine in the AP projection demonstrates a composite measured T-score from L1 through L4 of -1.7 representing osteopenia.

Scanning of the right proximal femur demonstrates osteopenia with the lowest T-score at the femoral neck at -2.3.

Scanning of the left proximal femur demonstrates osteopenia with the lowest T-score at the femoral neck at -2.4.

IMPRESSION:
Osteopenia as quantified above.

D: Jul 28 2005 5:51P T: Jul 29 2005 9:21A DPC

Trans By:
Dictated By: DPC: Jul 29 2005 9:21A
Dictation signed by: MARCHELLO BARBARISI M.D.: Jul 28 2005 5:51P
                      MARCHELLO BARBARISI M.D.: Jul 29 2005 2:11P

DXA scan report

healthy thirty-five-year-old woman. If your T-score falls between –1 and –2.5, you have mild bone loss called osteopenia. If your T score is –2.5 or lower, then you have osteoporosis and a significant increased risk of fractures. You can also look at your Z-score, but it only tells you how you compare to a similarly matched group of women your age and ethnic background. An eighty-year-old woman can have a normal Z-score even if she has severe osteoporosis.

I often have women tell me their DXA scan results are normal, yet when I look at the actual reports, I find that their Z-scores are normal but their T-scores are low so they need counseling about prevention of further bone loss. As you've heard me say before, get a copy of your report and learn what your results mean for you!

Now you know how to keep your preventive health care current as you celebrate each benchmark birthday. Of course, a lot more happens during your adult decades than just the tests and exams you get once a year or so. Part II, which is next on our agenda, is an intimate guide to the joys and challenges of the seasons of your life.

PART II

The Seasons of Your Life

4
Coming of Age

A Period Piece

IN THIS CHAPTER

- How We Become Females Before We're Born

- Puberty

- How Your Period Is Supposed to Work

- Dealing with Your Period

- Problems with Your Periods

According to an Apache legend, the goddess called Changing Woman represents the life cycle of women. She continually morphs from a child to a fertile woman to an ancient sage. Like other Native American nations, Apaches believe that women are powerful because they "bleed without dying." Each Apache girl celebrates her "first blood" during a four-day ceremony that opens with wise elders educating her about her sacred sexuality—the "fire within"—and culminates in a dance from dusk to sunrise. The tribal conviction is that while the girl is dancing, she embodies Changing Woman and therefore channels the goddess's power. As dawn colors the sky, both the male and female celebrants sing this song:

> *"Now you are entering the world.*
> *You will become an adult with responsibilities.*
> *Walk with honor and dignity.*
> *Be strong!"*

What a positive message that ritual sends about the menarche! In stark contrast, some cultures have traditionally banished women to menstrual huts each month until their flow has stopped. This practice continues in certain places around the world today. For that matter, in our own society "the curse" is still pretty much a taboo topic. There is, however, a burgeoning movement that encourages families to honor their daughters with "Red Parties" as they come of age. I think I would have loved that. I remember feeling grown up and special when I got my first period. I was so excited because several of my girlfriends had gotten theirs before I did and I had finally joined their ranks. On some level I knew even then that a woman's body is a wonder of nature that should be respected and admired. Much later in medical school when I learned how female anatomy is formed and functions, I was more in awe than ever. Unless you're a health-care professional yourself, you were probably taught nothing more than basic information about the mechanics of menstruation. That amounts to getting to the theater in the middle of the movie, so to speak. The story of the miracle of becoming a woman actually begins at conception. I'm going to let you in on how the process unfolds.

HOW WE BECOME FEMALES
BEFORE WE'RE BORN

I think most people know that X and Y chromosomes determine sex, but an informal survey of my friends and patients showed me that they weren't exactly sure what happens. Here's the scoop. Some sperm carry a Y, or male, chromosome and others carry an X, or female, chromosome. However, every egg, or ovum, has only an X chromosome. When one lucky sperm wins the race up the fallopian tube and penetrates an ovum, the result is a zygote. If the victorious sperm was carrying a Y chromosome, the zygote is destined to be a boy because the cell has an X chromosome from Mom and a Y chromosome from Dad. If the speediest sperm was carrying an X chromosome, the zygote is a girl-to-be, with an

X from Mom and an X from Dad. (So much for Henry VIII blaming his wives for failing to give him a son!)

The zygote makes the trip back down the fallopian tube in five days, during which time it divides into a ball of cells called a blastocyst. On about day six, the blastocyst implants into the lining of the uterus, the endometrium, which is rich with nourishing blood at that point in the menstrual cycle. At two weeks the blastocyst's inner group of cells becomes the embryo and the outer group becomes the placenta.

In the sixth week, limb buds appear when embryonic cells take on specific functions. During this process, called "differentiation," the embryo officially becomes a fetus. There are no visible anatomical differences between males and females at this point, but by seven weeks a fetus has the beginnings of what will make up the urinary and reproductive systems. Primitive structures called the genital tubercle, the urogenital groove and sinus, and the labioscrotal folds will develop into male or female organs. Genes are already being turned on or off to determine how the presence or amount of certain hormones will influence the evolution of these organs in males and females.

One of the hormones is testosterone and the other is the anti-Müllerian hormone (AMH). Both male and female fetuses start out with Wolffian and Müllerian ductal systems. These systems are named after the eighteenth-century German scientists who discovered them, Caspar Friedrich Wolff and Johann Peter Müller. The Wolffian ducts contribute to the development of the urinary tract in all fetuses but an infusion of testosterone in male fetuses gives rise to the uniquely masculine version while a lower level of testosterone dictates the development of the feminine version.

The male's generous supply of testosterone also programs the Wolffian ducts to develop into male reproductive organs. At the same time in males, the anti-Müllerian hormone inhibits the development of the Müllerian ducts so that they eventually wither and disappear. Females,

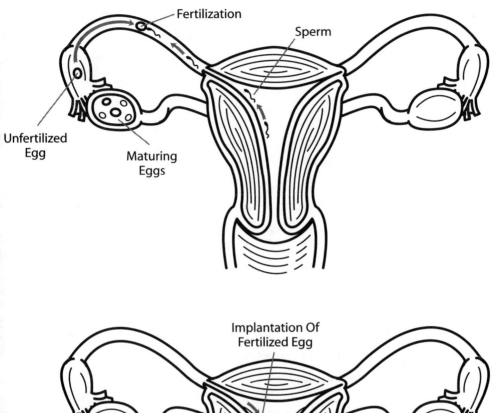

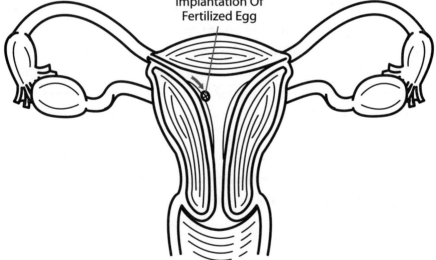

Fertilization

on the other hand, don't produce the anti-Müllerian hormone. Their Müllerian ducts go on to develop into the female reproductive system while their Wolffian ducts, having completed their task of creating the urinary system, gradually degenerate. Scientists call the female fetus's journey the "standard" or "default" action as if it weren't absolutely incredible!

At about ten weeks, a female fetus has her ovaries and all the eggs she'll ever make. Fetal ovaries produce the potent estrogen called estradiol, which helps the follicles that house the eggs begin to mature. However, estrogen plays almost no part in other aspects of prenatal sexual differentiation because maternal estrogen bathes the fetuses of both sexes.

PUBERTY

People tend to think of the menarche as the beginning of female puberty but a girl actually hits puberty two or three years before she gets her first period. On average, the menarche happens at about age thirteen. This means that the typical age for the start of female puberty is about ten. Puberty ends about three years after the first period, usually age sixteen, when the bony growth plates close and the female reproductive system is mature.

We all remember the growing pains, emotional and physical, of that time of life. As I said, I was thrilled when I got my first period. However, I wasn't so happy about my acne. I was also dying to have breasts big enough to fit into a bra. I remember leaving magazines around the house open to pages with pictures of training bras in hopes that my mom would get the hint!

On average, girls begin the process of puberty about one to two years earlier than boys and end it earlier as well. Remember how much more mature you thought you were than the boys in middle school? Well, you were!

THE STAGES OF PUBERTY

Hormonal Signals from the Adrenal Glands

The kick-off for puberty in both boys and girls happens with rising levels of the male hormone testosterone, an androgen from the adrenal glands. One result is the increased secretion of oil, or sebum, that can lead to acne. (See below for more about how androgens contribute to the signs of puberty.)

Hormonal Signals from the Hypothalamus

The next step happens when a region of the brain called the hypothalamus sends out pulses of hormones that stimulate the gonads. In males, the gonads are the testes and in females the gonads are the ovaries. The gonadotropin-releasing hormone (GnRH) comes first. As the name implies, it causes the pituitary gland to release luteinizing hormone (LH) and follicle-stimulating hormone (FSH). LH and FSH direct the ovaries to produce a variety of other hormones including steroid sex hormones, estradiol, and a little testosterone. (See the sidebar on pages 130–31 for the full list.) These hormones lead to changes in the brain, bones, muscles, skin, breasts, and reproductive organs.

THE SIGNS OF PUBERTY

Breast Buds

The first physical sign of puberty in girls is usually a firm, tender lump under the center of the nipple of one or both breasts. These are called breast buds and they occur on average at about age ten and a half. According to the widely used Tanner staging of puberty developed by the British pediatrician James Tanner, this is stage two of breast development. Stage one is the flat, prepubertal breast. Within six to twelve months after the buds appear, the swelling begins to soften and can be felt and seen extending beyond the edges of the nipple. This is stage three of breast development. After twelve more months the breasts reach stage four,

Why Do Different Girls Reach Puberty at Different ages?

Statistics show that more and more girls are going into puberty early, in particular African-American girls. Given the dramatic increase in childhood obesity, one theory is that the estrogen produced by the extra fat cells in girls who are overweight may be responsible for this trend toward "precocious puberty." There is also some evidence that water supplies contaminated with hormones and other substances from discarded medications and household products may cause girls to mature early. In addition, studies have shown that growing up in a dysfunctional house-hold may play a role is speeding up puberty.

Conversely, menarche may be slightly later when a girl grows up in a large family with a biological father present. Finally, girls with the eating disorders anorexia nervosa and bulimia may not reach the so-called "critical weight" of about 103 pounds that is necessary for periods to begin. When that happens, the menarche is delayed.

which is their mature size and shape. There is, of course, tremendous variation in the sizes and shapes of adult breasts and nipples.

Body Hair

Androgens contribute to pubic hair, underarm hair, and facial hair such as that annoying little mustache you have to bleach or wax. Pubic hair usually shows up within a few months after the breast buds. The first pubic hairs typically grow along the labia. This is Tanner stage two. Stage one is the lack of pubic hair in childhood. Stage three is usually reached within another six to twelve months when the hairs are too numerous to count and appear on the mons pubis (see chapter 1). By stage four, the hairs fill the pubic area. Stage five refers to the spread of pubic hair to the inner thighs and sometimes upward towards the navel. (This hair growth has kept waxing salons busy!)

Body Odor

The awakening of the ovaries during puberty causes changes in the fatty acid composition of sweat, which in turn causes body odor. It's usually an unpleasant smell and that's why you need a deodorant.

Maturing of the Reproductive Organs

Prior to the first period, the uterus and ovaries gradually increase in size. The surface lining of the vagina wakes up and changes in response to increasing levels of estrogen. It becomes thicker and a deeper pink in color. Whitish secretions that some girls describe as a discharge are a normal occurrence. These secretions usually continue throughout the fertile years and should not be confused with discharges that accompany some vaginal disorders (see chapter 7).

Menstrual Bleeding

The first menstrual bleeding typically occurs about two years after the appearance of the breast buds. The menstrual periods are not always regular during the first two years after the menarche. Ovulation is necessary for fertility, but it may not start right away.

Widening of the Pelvis

During this time, also in response to rising levels of estrogen, the lower half of the pelvis widens to allow the vagina to expand as a birth canal large enough for a baby when the time comes.

Increase in the Percentage of Fat

Fat tissue in females increases to a greater percentage of the total composition of the body than in males. The typical female distribution of fat

What Are the Major Hormones That Trigger Puberty?

- GnRH (gonadotropin-releasing hormone) is a protein hormone released from the hypothalamus that stimulates the cells of the anterior pituitary that produce LH and FSH.

- LH (luteinizing hormone) is a larger protein hormone secreted by the pituitary gland. The main target of LH is the cells of the ovaries. LH secretion changes more dramatically with the initiation of puberty than FSH does. LH levels increase about twenty-five fold with the onset of puberty compared with the two-and-a-half fold increase of FSH.

- FSH (follicle-stimulating hormone) is another protein hormone secreted by the cells of the pituitary. The main target of FSH is the ovarian follicles.

- Testosterone, the main androgen hormone, is produced in the ovaries and the adrenal gland and a small amount is produced from fat. It's an anabolic steroid. "Anabolic" comes from the Greek word meaning "to build up." Testosterone acts on androgen receptors throughout the body in both men and women to build up cellular tissue, especially muscles.

- Adrenal androgens are other steroids produced by the adrenal gland. They contribute to the androgenic events of early puberty in girls, such as the growth of body hair. The major adrenal androgens are dehydroepiandrosterone (DHEAS) and androstenedione, the building blocks of testosterone, and dehydroepiandrosterone sulfate, which is present in large amounts in the blood. (See chapter 2, page 33 for information about testosterone and reduced libido.)

- Estradiol, the principal human estrogen, is a steroid hormone produced from testosterone. (This strikes me as being like Eve made from Adam's rib by God). Estradiol acts on estrogen receptors throughout the body. The largest amounts of estradiol are produced by the ovaries with much lesser amounts coming from the adrenal glands and fat.

- IGF1 (insulin-like growth factor 1) rises substantially during puberty in response to increasing levels of the growth hormone and may be the principal mediator of the pubertal growth spurt. This hormone had not been identified when I was in medical school but it is now considered vital to healthy puberty.

- Leptin is a protein hormone produced by adipose or fat tissue. The leptin level seems to inform the brain how much adipose tissue there is in order to regulate the appetite and energy metabolism. It also plays a role in initiating the menarche, which usually will not begin until an adequate body fat mass has been achieved.

is in the breasts, hips, buttocks, thighs, upper arms, and mons pubis. Progressive differences in fat distribution as well as sex differences in local skeletal growth contribute to the typical female body shape by the end of puberty. At age ten the average girl has 6 percent more body fat than the average boy, but by the end of puberty, the average difference is nearly 50 percent. (See chapter 10 for more information about female fat.)

HOW YOUR PERIOD IS SUPPOSED TO WORK

PHASE ONE

The pituitary gland is the master command control center of the body's hormone and glandular systems. It's situated at the base of the brain behind the eyes. At the start of a normal menstrual cycle, the pituitary releases FSH into the bloodstream. When the FSH reaches the ovaries, where immature ova are waiting, it stimulates one egg and the follicles around it so that they develop. Sometimes more than one egg develops. That's what leads to the possibility of fraternal twins or other multiples. The follicular cells surrounding the egg or eggs begin to produce estrogen once they've been stimulated by FSH.

PHASE TWO

Around the middle of the cycle, the pituitary gland produces LH. This hormone causes the cells on the surface of the ovary to break open and release the egg. After the egg is released, the ovary begins to produce progesterone, the other main female hormone, along with estrogen. If you become pregnant, the ovaries continue to make these hormones for about three months until the placenta is able to take over hormone production for both itself and the developing fetus. (This LH surge is the basis of many over-the-counter ovulation tests. When you test positive in urine for LH surge, ovulation will occur in about twelve hours or so.)

PHASE THREE

If you don't become pregnant, the ovaries stop making progesterone about two weeks after ovulation. Without this hormone, the uterine lining cells can't survive. They die and are shed as the menstrual flow. It is the sudden cessation of hormone production that leads to your period. (See chapter 5, page 145, for an explanation of how birth control pills mimic this process.) Typically the flow goes on for about four days. Then the cycle, usually lasting about twenty-eight days, starts all over again.

DEALING WITH YOUR PERIOD

At the beginning of this chapter, I waxed rhapsodic about the beauty of the Apache menarche celebration and its positive message of empowerment for women because we "bleed without dying." Nevertheless, dealing for forty-odd years with a periodic flow of blood over which we have no control is probably not high up on any woman's list of pleasurable

Are Menstrual Cycles Really in Tune with the Moon?

Although the word "menstruation" and "moon" are both derived from the Greek and Latin words for "month," we have no scientific evidence that menstrual cycles are affected by the phases of the moon in the way that ocean tides are. The idea that menstruation is related to the moon probably came from the ancient lunar calendars that had twelve months of twenty-eight days each. However, the moon's cycle actually lasts twenty-nine and a half days. There are now over forty calendars used in cultures and religions around the world with months of varying lengths. The most popular is the one we use in the United States, a solar version called the Gregorian calendar because it was initiated in 1592 during the time of Pope Gregory XIII. All of that notwithstanding, the notion of a connection between menstrual cycles and the moon's phases persists, especially in shamanism and witchcraft.

activities! We have anal sphincters and urinary sphincters that communicate with the brain in order to shut tight until we are in a safe place to eliminate stool and urine. However, the vaginal muscles don't get any neural messages that would allow us to choose when to pass menstrual blood. True, as you'll learn in chapters 8 and 9, anal and urinary sphincters don't always work as they should. The point, though, is that they are designed to put us in command of those bodily functions.

Scientists don't know why a similar system isn't in place for menstruation. However, a somewhat tongue-in-cheek 1995 article by J. D. Gillies, M.D., in the highly respected *British Medical Journal* suggests that "the present human form is the first draft of a cosmic design." Dr. Gillies goes on to give a list "respectfully submitted to the Almighty" of organs and functions that could use some improvement in future

Accidents Happen

Just about every woman has a period "horror story"! Here are a few from my patients and friends:

Madison, Age 22

"I got my period for the first time in the middle of my ballet recital when I was twelve. I was wearing a white tutu and pink tights and I saw the blood when I bent forward for a step called a 'reverence.' I thought I would die of embarrassment but I was trained that the show must go on so I didn't leave the stage. I made it through the rest of that dance before I ran back to the dressing room. Another girl gave me a tampon and clean tights. I put on my next costume and went back out to do the butterfly dance. When I told my teacher that I had made my next entrance on time in spite of the accident, she said, 'Well, I should hope so!' Ballet teachers are tough! My mother just said, 'Welcome to the club, kiddo.'"

Jessica, Age 38

"This happened last year right after I made partner at the law firm where I work. The other partners gave me a party after work and I had to make a little speech. I was nervous because I was the first female partner and all the guys were a lot older. They proposed a toast. I stood up and felt a gush. My period wasn't due for another week! I guess the stress brought it on. Luckily I was wearing a skirt instead of a pantsuit. My speech was short and sweet and I made it to the bathroom before anything ran down my leg!"

Laura, Age 45

"My periods started getting irregular about three years ago so I figured I was going into perimenopause. The unpredictability drove me crazy. When I did get my period, it would be like this sudden hemorrhage. So one day when I was in the stands watching my son's soccer game, my period came and my jeans were totally soaked. I had a coat with me that I had taken off earlier when the sun got hot so I put the coat on and headed for the ladies' room. I had learned to carry super tampons with me all the time. I drove home and changed into a clean pair of jeans. When I went back to pick up Scot, I asked one of my friends to fill me in on what had happened during the game. She said I didn't miss anything. Our team lost anyway!"

models. Among the "defects" on Dr. Gilles's list is the fact that "the vagina, unlike the rectum, is not equipped with a watertight sphincter, so incontinence of menstrual flow is a constant worry." He commiserates with us because "a woman spends nearly 20 percent of her time between thirteen and fifty coping with bleeding." Fortunately, we have an arsenal of products to help us do just that:

- Disposable pads. Absorbent "sanitary napkins" have sticky strips for attaching to your underwear. They come in a variety of sizes, shapes, and absorbencies, with and without "wings," for use during times of light and heavy flow as well as overnight. During the day change your pad at least every three or four hours even if the flow is light. Also don't wear panty liners twenty-four/seven. (See chapter 7, page 212 for information about preventing vaginal infections.)
- Reusable pads. Available at health food stores and online, these "green" alternatives can be washed and worn again. They come with clips.

- Tampons. These are the familiar tubes of absorbent material that you insert into the vagina. If you're a teenager new to tampons, follow the directions on the package about how to insert and remove them or have your mom or a girlfriend teach you. I remember a bunch of us girls in the restroom at school with one leg up on the toilet seat bracing ourselves as we tried to put in a tampon. Practice makes perfect! Sliding the tampon in and out is easy unless you have a medical problem (see chapter 7, page 228). You can use a tampon even if you're a virgin. The tampon won't "pop your cherry," but it may stretch your hymen. This causes no harm. Be sure to change your tampon every four to six hours. Leaving tampons in too long can lead to a dangerous bacterial infection called toxic shock syndrome.
- Menstrual cups. These are made of flexible materials such as rubber or silicone. They catch the menstrual flow. You need to empty them and wash them although some models are disposable. They look something like a diaphragm but they are not a method of contraception and they do not protect against STIs.

PROBLEMS WITH YOUR PERIODS

PREMENSTRUAL SYNDROME (PMS)

An estimated 80 percent of women experience one or two symptoms of PMS at least every now and then. However, some women have several symptoms every month for years and others have a version of PMS that's so severe it has its own name as a psychiatric diagnosis: "premenstrual dysphoric disorder" (PMDD). "Dysphoria," by the way, means a general "blue" feeling or a pervasive unhappiness.

There are no diagnostic tests for PMS or PMDD. Doctors rely on what patients tell them about symptoms. If you think you have PMS or PMDD, be sure to keep a health journal (see chapter 3)! Treatments range from simple lifestyle changes such as exercise and adequate sleep to medical intervention with antidepressants or hormone therapy. The options that are right for you depend on whether your condition is mild, tolerable, or disabling. Typical symptoms include:

- mood swings, including anxiety and dysphoria
- bloating
- cramps
- insomnia
- headaches
- acne
- skin rashes
- susceptibility to eye infections such as conjunctivitis

DYSMENORRHEA

This refers to extremely painful periods. Primary dysmenorrhea has no underlying cause and it usually subsides after the teens and twenties. Secondary dysmenorrhea is a symptom, not a disease in itself. The cause could be conditions such as fibroids, endometriosis, or ovarian cysts (see chapter 7 for more information). As always, keep a health journal so that you can help your doctor make a diagnosis.

MENORRHAGIA

This refers to extremely heavy periods. As with secondary dysmenorrhea, it typically has an underlying cause such as fibroids or endometriosis. Menopausal women often experience menorrhagia during the time that their cycles are becoming unpredictable (see chapter 6, page 189). Keep a health journal and see a doctor.

AMENORRHEA

This refers to the absence of periods. Primary amenorrhea is the term used when a girl hasn't had her menarche by the age of sixteen. She may have structural or chromosomal abnormalities and should go to a doctor for an evaluation. Secondary amenorrhea happens when a girl or woman has been menstruating but suddenly stops. I was taught in medical school that unsuspected pregnancy is the number one cause of secondary amenorrhea, so be on the lookout for it. Also, extremely low body weight and excessive exercise are often the culprits. Most girls and women with eating disorders end up with amenorrhea. Other causes could be hormonal imbalances and thyroid malfunction. *Warning:* Continue to use contraception if you don't want to get pregnant. You may still be ovulating or you may suddenly begin ovulating again. In any case, keep a health journal and see a doctor.

Now you know all about how you developed as a female from your time in the womb to your passage through puberty. The whole point of the maturing of your reproductive organs is, of course, to prepare your body for pregnancy. Yet for all of us, whether and when we want to be pregnant is a very personal matter. In the next chapter I'll give you information to help you take charge of the fertile years of your life.

5

For unto You a Child Could Be Born

Charting Your Course

IN THIS CHAPTER

- Birth Control Basics: Considering the Options

- Trying Can Be Trying: Fertility and Infertility Explained

- Great with Child: Pregnancy and Childbirth

- Oh, Baby! Your Body, Your Emotions, and Your Life as a Mom

People have been practicing some form of birth control since the dawn of recorded history and probably before then. An ancient Egyptian papyrus dating from about 1500 B.C. has instructions for making an herbal contraceptive suppository. The Greeks and Romans relied on herbs as well, in particular a form of fennel called silphium that was so popular it became extinct. On the other hand, fertility rites and prayers have also always been part of cultures around the world. Brides in Ancient Rome carried symbolic sheaves of wheat, early Europeans did a ritual maypole dance, and the Catholic Church has a prayer to St. Gerard to "beseech the Master of life from whom all paternity proceedeth to render me fruitful in offspring."

In other words, "family planning," that often controversial and politically charged aspect of modern life, is nothing new. Like women since time immemorial, at various points in your life, you may want to postpone getting pregnant, or yearn to have a child, or try to space your pregnancies, or not want to be pregnant ever again—or ever.

Fortunately, thanks to modern medicine and current laws that give you unprecedented reproductive freedom, you have more options for taking charge of your fertile years than was true even a generation ago. Whether you're a teen who has only recently joined the company of women or a twenty- to forty-something, the information that follows will get you up to speed.

(Pssst. If you're past the childbearing years yourself, don't skip this chapter. You'll learn what's different for the younger women in your life compared to the status quo back when you were their age. However, you'll also see that important facets of fertility, pregnancy, and childbirth haven't changed at all. Neither has the reality of those first weeks of motherhood when the sleep-deprived new mom may feel as though her personhood is slipping away. I can almost guarantee that in the role of grandmother—or great aunt or even close family friend—you'll be wanted and needed along the way as the voice of experience. That will be true whether you're down the block or visiting by e-mail and Web cam, so stay in the loop!)

BIRTH CONTROL BASICS: CONSIDERING THE OPTIONS

NATURAL METHODS

Abstinence

This is a no-brainer. If you don't have sex, you won't get pregnant. (You can't get pregnant from toilet seats!) The catch, of course, is that unless you're in a nunnery, your chances of remaining chaste are probably pretty low. Even teens who take virginity pledges, often in elaborate ceremonies mimicking debutante balls and involving a promise ring from Daddy, are statistically highly likely to break their celibacy vows well before they walk down the aisle. One study released in 2008 that had tracked over 900 American teenagers found no differences among pledgers and non-pledgers regarding the frequency of premarital sex. In fact, 84 percent of the 289 teens in the study who originally said they had made a virginity pledge later denied that they had ever done so. This is why I'm opposed to so-called "abstinence-only" sex education. Our children deserve to know how to protect themselves not only from unplanned pregnancies but from STIs. And, no, teaching them about what I call "Smart Sex" won't make them any more or less likely to "go all the way" (see chapter 2). However, if you're an adult, the choice of whether or not to be abstinent is up to you—and to your partner if you have one. Depending on how important not getting pregnant is at any time in your life, you may in fact want to opt for this method since it's the only one that's absolutely fail-safe!

Outercourse

This term made it into the Merriam-Webster dictionary back in 1986 but the American Heritage Dictionary didn't list it until 2000. For you boomers in the audience, outercourse is not unlike "necking," "petting," and "making out"—activities that were usually engaged in at the drive-in or elsewhere in a parked car where you hoped not to be discovered. There are differences, however. The list of what most couples used to do was limited to kissing, French kissing, and—for the daring—fondling of breasts and genitals. Today's teens may add oral and anal sex as well as "dry humping" (rubbing genitals on genitals without penetration) and mutual masturbation. As the Planned Parenthood Web site warns, "sperm may come into contact with the vagina," and "some people may find it hard to abstain from intercourse." No kidding! I'll add to that the fact that oral and anal sex carry with them the risk of STIs including HPV infections that can cause cervical, oral, tonsillar, and anal cancer (see chapter 2, page 39). Overall, counting on outercourse to prevent pregnancy, however trendy the concept may be, is a very bad idea as far as I'm concerned.

Fertility Awareness Methods (FAM)

Also called natural family planning (NFP), FAM involves several procedures for determining when a woman is ovulating. The goal is to time intercourse in order to prevent or achieve a pregnancy. One of the techniques is the rhythm method that has long been approved by the Catholic Church. This system has been dubbed "Vatican Roulette" because charting the phases of a menstrual cycle by using a calendar alone is definitely dicey. Newer techniques that are somewhat more reliable include testing the cervical mucus and keeping track of basal body temperature. The Catholic Church approves of these. People practicing FAM for birth control need to abstain for nine days of the month including the days just before and after ovulation to account for how long eggs and sperm can live. Since many of us prefer not to have sex when we're menstruating, either because of cramps or because the prospect is so messy, that only leaves two weeks out of the month when a FAM couple can make love. Another drawback is that FAM offers no protection against STIs. However, if you and your partner are in a monogamous relationship and you're both committed to ensuring that the method works because it's the only one acceptable to you, you may have a pretty decent rate of success. Remember, though, that periods become more unpredictable as you approach menopause. That's the reason for late-in-life "menopause babies." I come from a French Catholic family and my mother was pregnant with my youngest brother, her eighth child, at my older sister's wedding.

Lactational Amenorrhea Method (LAM)

Primitive and rural societies often relied on breastfeeding to space pregnancies because ovulation is usually suppressed while a woman is lactating. The Catholic Church approves of this method. However, current research shows that for this method to be effective, you have to be breastfeeding exclusively or supplementing with other liquids or foods only every now and then. Official guidelines also say that after the baby is six months old, you need another form of contraception even if you're not menstruating yet because ovulation may start again. I can attest to the fact that ovulation might start even earlier than that. I was nursing my newborn first son when I got pregnant for the second time. My physician father-in-law, whom we were visiting at the time, sent my urine sample to a laboratory. He reported back that I was going to have "Irish

What Is The "Morning-After Pill"?

Plan B, the FDA-approved emergency oral contraceptive, has high doses of a synthetic hormone that's in birth control pills. You need to take the first pill no later than seventy-two hours (three days) after you've had unprotected sex. The earlier you take the pill, the better the chance that it will work. You also need to take a second pill twelve hours after the first one. The first pill acts to suppress ovulation and the second pill stops the sperm from traveling up the fallopian tubes. However, Plan B will not end an existing pregnancy so don't confuse emergency contraception with medical abortion (see the "Abortion" section, below).

You can buy Plan B over the counter if you're eighteen or older and you have proof of your age. If you're younger than that, you need a doctor's prescription. Be aware that Plan B has side effects such as nausea, headaches, cramping, and heavy bleeding and that it's only 80 percent effective even if taken as directed. Also, it doesn't protect against STIs. Once again, let me wag my finger and remind you that smart women like you should practice Smart Sex! Certainly, if you've been the victim of rape or if your partner's condom broke or came off when he pulled out, the morning-after pill may be a godsend. But please don't let one too many margaritas or a sudden surge of mutual passion put you in a situation you could have avoided!

twins," a popular reference to siblings born close together. Not long after that, we learned that I was actually going to have what might be called "Irish triplets" since I was in fact carrying twins! I love all three of my boys dearly, but those first few years were hectic to say the least.

Withdrawal

Teenagers have probably always known about "pulling out." The timing, of course, has to be exquisitely accurate and no semen or even pre-ejaculate can get onto or into the vagina. Practiced without a condom, this method invites the swapping of STIs. If you get carried away and neither one of you thought to bring a condom, withdrawal is your best bet. But next time, remember the Girl Scout motto and "Be prepared"!

HORMONAL CONTRACEPTIVES
The Pill

I have taken oral contraceptives at both ends of my menstrual life first as a young woman for birth control and later as a mature woman to manage my erratic and often heavy periods. (There's more about my perimenopausal experience in chapter 6.) As for my initial use of the Pill, I was a first-year nursing student at the Hospital of the University of Pennsylvania in 1967, seven years after the Pill was introduced and shortly after changes in state laws allowed physicians and health centers to prescribe the Pill without regard to age or marital status. I wasn't even sexually active but since everybody else was taking the Pill, I wanted it, too, "just in case." My friends and I never considered any downside other than the need to see a doctor to get the prescription. The cost was $15 or less a month back then. I remember the gruff, aging doctor—a man, of course—behind his big, dark desk. He asked me a few questions about my medical history. There was no exam, no need to get undressed, just "Here is your prescription" and I was out the door. Believe it or not, the dose of estrogen, a whopping 150 µg (micrograms), was at least seven times greater than the amount in pills that are currently dispensed. The

How Do Birth Control Pills Work?

The reason you don't get pregnant when you're on the Pill is that doses of progestin (a synthetic version of progesterone) and estrogen work together to suppress or turn off the ovaries, thicken the cervical mucus to inhibit the movement of sperm, and alter the uterine lining so implantation won't take place even if fertilization does manage to occur.

There is one natural oral progesterone, Prometrium, for post-menopausal women. It is "micronized" so stomach acid won't destroy it. However, when the Pill was developed and tested, this product was not yet available. Drug companies continue to use synthetic compounds for birth control pills because the progestin has a history of success in preventing pregnancies. It causes more side effects than naturally produced progesterone does (such as acne, depression, bloating, headaches), but the newer versions, Yaz and Yasmin, have been modified with a newer progestin to mitigate those problems. However, we still don't have as much long-term data on the safety of these products as we do for the older Pill combinations.

As for why you get a period when you're on the Pill, albeit typically a light one, the mechanism is the same as the natural one I explained back in chapter 4. When you're not on the Pill, your menstrual flow starts as soon as your production of estrogen and progesterone stops because you didn't get pregnant that month. An abrupt end to hormones is also what triggers your flow when you're taking combination birth control pills. Seven of the pills in the twenty-eight day pack are placebos (sugar pills) with no hormones. If you have a twenty-one-day pack, you stop taking pills for seven days. The effect is the same either way. The only reason the placebos are included in the twenty-eight-day pack is to keep you in the habit of taking a pill every day. (See "Mini-Pill," page 148, for information about progestin-only pills.)

new, lower doses have greatly reduced the health risks associated with taking the Pill. Today we can use oral contraceptives not only for birth control but also to treat acne, deal with PCOS (see chapter 7, page 224), manage severe cramps, reduce ovarian cysts, minimize blood loss and anemia, and even help reduce the risk of ovarian cancer.

The Pill is 97 percent effective as a contraceptive if taken as directed and 92 percent effective even if a couple of pills are missed. Some women find that when they stop taking the Pill, their bodies need a few months to get back on a regular cycle. However, the Pill will not make you infertile. Most women age forty and under (or thirty-five and under for smokers) can safely take oral contraceptives. (The guidelines for the perimenopausal years are different. See chapter 6.) Even so, I want you to know about possible complications:

- Phlebitis. Also called thrombophlebitis, this refers to blood clots. They usually occur in the legs. Serious complications include clots that travel to the lungs and cause pulmonary embolisms, and clots that can cause heart attacks and strokes. The risk of phlebitis is now fairly low. However, if you smoke and are over the age of thirty-five, absolutely do not take oral contraceptives—your risk is too high. Other risk factors for phlebitis include family history of blood-clotting disorder, obesity, prior phlebitis or blood clots, a sedentary lifestyle, and immobility such as after surgery or when you're in a wheelchair or have a cast on your leg.
- Heart disease and stroke. Besides blood clots, another cause of heart problems and strokes related to taking the Pill may be a buildup of plaque in the arteries, but this probably only occurs in women who take the Pill for ten years or more. This was the finding in a recent study from Belgium.
- High blood pressure. A slight rise in blood pressure is common but it's not a big concern unless your pressure was elevated in the first place.

If I'm under Thirty-Five and I Smoke, Can I Take the Pill?

Many doctors do prescribe the Pill for smokers under the age of thirty-five. I think that's crazy but others say it's justified when there is simply no way a girl or young woman will stop smoking and her chances of an unwanted pregnancy are high because she's not committed to using other forms of birth control consistently. If that describes you, think twice about accepting a prescription for the Pill. As always, you are the only one who can decide what risks you're willing to take. Also, smoking is a killer in other ways as well. You know what I'm going to say next, don't you? Find a way to kick the habit! There are cessation programs and support groups that can help you. Do yourself and your loved ones as favor by conquering your addiction to cigarettes. You can succeed!

- Breast cancer. Long-term use of the Pill causes a slight increase in the risk of breast cancer although the risk of ovarian and endometrial cancer is actually reduced. The risk of breast cancer remains slightly elevated in the first nine years after stopping the Pill. Since the overall risk of breast cancer in young women is fortunately small, this increase in risk does little to dissuade most women from taking the Pill. However, doctors may counsel women who inherit the BRCA 1 or 2 genes or have a strong family history of breast cancer not to take the Pill, although this is not an across-the-board contraindication. (See chapter 3, page 114.)
- Bloating, weight gain, breast tenderness, headaches, reduced libido, and mood swings. These symptoms are not serious health risks but many women can't tolerate them. My suggestion is to stick with the

regimen for at least a few months because the problems may lessen or go away as your body gets accustomed to the hormone doses.

Mini-Pill

Progestin-only Pills, often called mini-Pills, are better for breastfeeding women than combination Pills because estrogen can limit the milk supply. Mini-Pills may also be safer for women over thirty-five. Some women experience more nuisance symptoms such as bloating and mood swings than when they're on combination Pills, but others report less nausea and fewer headaches. Only you can tell whether the mini-Pill is an acceptable option for you. One drawback of the mini-Pill is that periods or spotting are irregular and unpredictable because you take hormones every day rather than stopping for seven days as you would with the combination Pill. Another potential problem is that you have to take the Pill at the same time every day. If you're even three hours late, you need to use another method of contraception for the next two days. If you miss a pill altogether, you're not protected for the rest of that month.

Extended-Range Oral Contraceptives

The traditional combination Pill mimics Mother Nature in that you bleed once a month even though the normal process of releasing an egg is suppressed. With the new extended-range pills marketed as Seasonale and Seasonique, you only get your period four times a year after your body adjusts to the regimen. That can take as long as a year, during which you'll have irregular periods and spotting. With the brand called Lybrel, you eventually have no periods at all. These options may appeal to some women for the obvious reason that you no longer have to deal with a monthly flow. On the other hand, you no longer have the monthly assurance that you're not pregnant. In fact the drug company that makes Lybrel recommends that you use a home pregnancy test kit every month just to be sure you're not among the small percentage of women for whom the product isn't fail-safe. Needless to say, this constitutes additional expense and is something of a bother. Beyond that, these products seem to me to involve a lot of manipulation of a woman's normal functioning and they deliver more hormones than the combination Pill does—perhaps more than is good for you—and definitely more than you need to avoid pregnancy, which is why you're taking the Pill in the first place. I will reserve judgment about the extended-range Pills until long-term studies of thousands of women assure me that these methods really are as safe and effective as traditional Pills and that there is no danger of problems later on, including infertility.

Transdermal Patch

In general I am a big fan of transdermal or "through the skin" delivery of hormones because they bypass the liver and thus prevent potential complications such as increased blood clotting and higher blood pressure. They even reduce the risk of gall bladder disease. Also, the patches for postmenopausal women allow for an overall lower dose of hormones. Unfortunately however, the only birth control patch available in the United States, Ortho Evra, delivers about 60 percent *more* estrogen into the bloodstream than oral contraceptives do and needs to be reformulated to lower the dose. (See chapter 6, page 183, for information about the safe and effective transdermal hormone patches available for postmenopausal women.)

Hormone Implants

Implanon is a rod about the size of a matchstick. A trained clinician implants the rod in your upper arm. The implant releases progestin and you are protected against pregnancy for up to three years. This low-maintenance method is 99 percent effective. The side effects and risks are similar to those for the progestin-only mini-Pill. Periods will be irregular and possibly heavy for the first six months to a year but then they may stop altogether. This is normal, and fertility returns not long after the implant is removed.

Hormone Injections

There is a shot of progestin called Depo-Provera that you can get every three months. However, Depo-Provera has been linked to low bone mass in the hip and spine, a condition called osteopenia that is a precursor of osteoporosis. Because we hit our maximum bone mass by age thirty-five and it is all downhill from there, no older woman—or any woman for that matter—can afford to lose more bone than occurs naturally with aging. However, recent studies suggest that bone loss can be reversed after you stop the Depo-Provera. If that proves to be true, Depo-Provera might make sense for a very young woman who is at high risk for unwanted pregnancy, because compliance—meaning remembering to take the Pill every day—might be a genuine problem for her.

Vaginal Birth Control Ring

A relatively new hormonal contraceptive option is the "combined contraceptive vaginal ring" or NuvaRing. It's a flexible transparent plastic ring that's very easy to insert. It can't get lost inside (see chapter 1, page 10). However, it does require strong pelvic muscles to hold it in, so you're not a good candidate for this method if you have pelvic prolapse, a condition in which the pelvic floor muscles are stretched and weakened. This can occur as a result of having a baby vaginally. Also, even if you have excellent control of your pelvic muscles, the ring occasionally comes out when you strain with a bowel movement, have sex, or remove a tampon. If you put the ring back in within three hours, it will still be effective. Be sure to rinse it first with lukewarm water. The ring releases only 15 mcg of ethinyl estradiol and 120 mcg of etonogestrel (progestin) per day. This is a way of getting systemic estrogen with fewer or none of the potential problems, such as blood clots and heart disease, that may be associated with oral contraceptives. You leave the ring in place for twenty-one consecutive days and then remove it for a seven-day interval to bring on a "withdrawal bleed." You insert a new ring for the next cycle. One disadvantage is that because the ring remains in the vagina for a full three weeks, you have a higher than normal risk of getting yeast vaginitis. The risk of bacterial vaginosis is actually reduced with the ring because more of the "good bacteria" called lactobacilli live in the vagina with the ring as a result of the increased estrogen level. (See chapter 7, page 200 to learn more about yeast infections and bacterial vaginosis.) The NuvaRing sounds to me like a good option but I'd like to see more research on systemic effects, safety, effectiveness, and patient satisfaction.

BARRIER CONTRACEPTIVES

All of these methods work by preventing the sperm from entering the cervix or from traveling up the fallopian tubes. Several of them are more effective if used along with spermicides. These are available as creams, gels, foam, and suppositories. Spermicides can also be used alone but that reduces their effectiveness. The only one of the barrier methods that protects against STIs is the condom.

Condoms

This is the familiar sheath for your partner's penis that protects against both pregnancy and STIs. See chapter 2 for complete information.

Female Condom

Again, this topic is fully covered in chapter 2.

Cervical Cap

This is a silicone cup that fits over the entrance to the cervix. If you've given birth vaginally, this is not a particularly effective method, and even if you've never been pregnant, the cap works only about 85 percent of the time. Using spermicide with the cap helps you get better results.

Diaphragm

This is a latex cup with a flexible rim. You insert the diaphragm so that it covers your cervix. Used correctly and consistently, a diaphragm is about 95 percent effective especially if you also use a spermicide. However, if you're prone to urinary tract infections (see chapter 9), this isn't the best option for you.

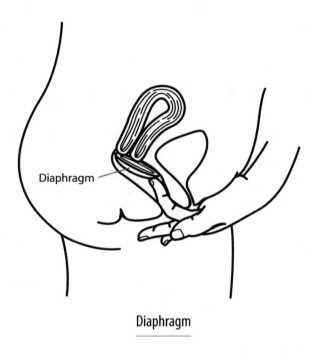

Diaphragm

Diaphragm

The Sponge

The only brand available is the Today Sponge. You can get it over the counter. The sponge is a round piece of foam that covers the cervix and releases a spermicide. It's easy to insert. You need to leave it in for six hours after sex but you shouldn't leave it in for longer than thirty hours. For women who have never given birth, the sponge is up to 90 percent effective. For women who have given birth, it's about 75 percent effective.

Intra-Uterine Device (IUD)

IUDs have been around since the 1970s and they have been improved since then. Birth control lore has it that the ancient Egyptians invented the first IUDs when they inserted pebbles into the uteruses of female camels so they wouldn't get pregnant during long trips through the desert! The devices are T-shaped and made of flexible plastic. A health-care provider inserts the IUD into your uterus, where it can stay for as long as five to twelve years. ParaGard IUDs contain copper, which impairs the sperms' ability to swim up the fallopian tubes. However, ParaGard IUDs can cause very heavy blood flow. Mirena IUDs contain progestin, which alters the mucous environment so that it's unfriendly for the sperm. This version actually lightens the monthly blood flow. Both types of IUDs are up to 99 percent effective and they can be used as emergency contraception if they're inserted within five days after unprotected sex.

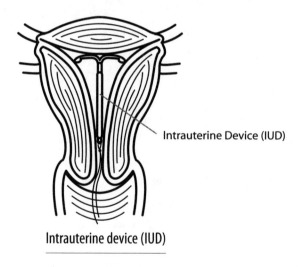

Intrauterine Device (IUD)

Intrauterine device (IUD)

ABORTION

Abortion is the termination of a pregnancy. Technically, the term refers to spontaneous abortion (commonly knows as miscarriage) as well as to induced abortion. However, we have come to use the term to mean induced abortion. Abortion up to twenty-four weeks into a pregnancy became legal in this country with the landmark Roe vs. Wade decision by the Supreme Court in 1973. However, abortion rights remain a contentious political issue to this day. Here are your options if you make the very personal decision to end a pregnancy.

Medical Abortion

The pills that terminate a pregnancy that's eight weeks or less along go by the brand name Mifeprex. An earlier name was RU486. You take one pill, mifepristone, in the doctor's office or at an abortion clinic. This blocks the production of the progesterone needed to support the pregnancy. Then twenty-four to seventy-two hours later while you're at home, you take a second pill called misoprostol. This causes uterine contractions so that you have a miscarriage. The process can take six to eight hours and sometimes more. You may experience nausea, vomiting, headaches, and very heavy bleeding and cramping. You'll go for a checkup two weeks later to make sure the process was completed. In about 5 percent of cases, there is still tissue in the uterus that has to be suctioned out. There is also an injection method of medical abortion using an experimental cancer treatment that stops cells from dividing. Medical abortion is an "off label" use of this drug and the procedure has not been tested long-term for safety and effectiveness.

Vacuum Suction Abortion

Also called aspiration, this is an in-clinic procedure that can be performed up to twelve weeks into pregnancy. You'll be given antibiotics to prevent infection and you'll be given pain medication. The health-care provider will insert a device into your uterus that will empty it. The procedure takes about ten or fifteen minutes once you have had a consultation and been given the medications. Sometimes an instrument called a curettage is used to ensure that all the tissue has been removed. This is called dilation and curettage (D&C). Nine out of ten surgical abortions in this country are this type, with or without a D&C.

Second Trimester Abortions

These are illegal unless the mother's life is at stake. If you want to terminate your pregnancy, please take action during the first trimester. One method of second trimester abortion is called dilation and evacuation (D&E) and the other involves the injection of a saline solution. Abortions after twenty-four weeks of pregnancy (the third trimester) when a fetus is considered viable outside the womb are illegal.

PERMANENT BIRTH CONTROL METHODS

Female Sterilization Methods

These are surgical procedures and they are often coupled with childbirth. Tubal ligation involves tying or cutting the fallopian tubes so that sperm can't make the trip up to find an egg for fertilization. You're protected immediately. Another procedure with the brand name Essure involves metal rings that are placed on the tubes. This causes scar tissue that blocks the path of the sperm. The process takes about three months, so use another form of birth control in the meantime. Sterilization is not reversible. However, in very rare cases the tubes may spontaneously reconnect so that there's a passage large enough to allow sperm to pass through but not large enough for a fertilized egg. The result could be an ectopic or tubal pregnancy. See your doctor if you have severe abdominal or shoulder pain, unexplained vaginal bleeding, or fainting spells.

Vasectomy

This is the male version of sterilization. The tube leading from each testicle is called a vas deferens. After sperm are made in the testicles, they pass through these tubes and mix with glandular material from the seminal vesicles and the prostate to become semen. That's the fluid that your partner ejaculates when he has an orgasm. During a vasectomy the tubes are clamped, cut, or sealed. After the procedure the patient will be asked to bring semen samples to a physician's office or laboratory for two- or three-month intervals so that tests can determine whether the sperm count is low enough to ensure that pregnancy won't occur. In 2008 the FDA approved an over-the-counter home testing kit called SpermCheck. A man who has had a vasectomy can still get an erection and experience orgasms but the semen he ejaculates won't have any or very much sperm in it. Complications of the procedures are extremely uncommon although infection can occur. The signs of infection are swelling at the site of the incision, blood or pus coming from the incision, and fever. Your partner should see a doctor if any of these symptoms occur. In rare cases the tubes can reconnect by themselves, and some attempts at surgical reconnection are successful. However, as with female sterilization, a vasectomy should be viewed as permanent.

If you're sure you've completed your family or you don't want to get pregnant at all, consider the permanent birth control options with great care. The idea of a divorce down the road may seem impossible now but the impossible does happen. Also, you could be widowed while you're still in your childbearing years. By the same token, your husband could become a widower. These scenarios are painful to contemplate but please have the courage to talk over every possibility before you close off future reproductive options for either you or your partner. However, many people who opt for permanent birth control are very glad they did so. In this country more women choose sterilization than men even though the procedure for men is simpler and safer. On the other hand, some fathers are happy to be the spouse who takes the step that will ensure worry-free (and condom-free!) sex and will guarantee that the family won't be stressed financially by more children. I think that's great. Let him take some responsibility for birth control after *you've* been dealing with it all these years!

That's the decision my husband and I made once we were blessed with three healthy, wonderful sons. I know how fortunate I was to reach that point in my life as a woman. I had my share of problems along the way and you'll read about them in detail in chapters 7, 8, and 9. For now I'll just say that all I had to deal with were nuisance conditions such as a huge hemorrhoid after giving birth, pain during sex the first time we made love after the baby was born, occasional vaginal infections, and some embarrassing urinary leaks because of stress incontinence. A lot of women have much bigger issues such as trouble getting pregnant, scary complications during pregnancy and childbirth, and difficulty with breastfeeding. But that list doesn't have to be as much of a downer as it sounds. Let's have a look at the ways you can cope physically and emotionally if you run up against obstacles on the way to motherhood and mothering.

TRYING CAN BE TRYING: FERTILITY AND INFERTILITY EXPLAINED

The teenage years are among the most fertile ones of a woman's life. That accounts for the fact that teens get pregnant so easily if they have unprotected sex or a condom breaks. Those incidents cause plenty of hand-wringing today. Yet centuries ago when the average life expectancy for women was decades lower than it is today, having babies early made sense. At this point in history, though, the majority of us want to wait until we're at least twenty-something or often well beyond that before we start a family. We hope to finish college and perhaps postgraduate work, take our time finding Mr. Right, get some traction in a career, and maybe put him through law school or med school or his MBA as well. Only then are we ready to "settle down" and become mothers. Unfortunately, our bodies haven't evolved to catch up with this plan. Female fertility starts declining when we're in our twenties. Imagine that! You've got a window of about ten years or less from the time your ovaries mature while you're in high school until your chances of conceiving begin to diminish. Not only that, but after the age of thirty-five, fertility drops even more rapidly and by forty-five a woman has a 1 percent chance of conceiving using her own eggs. Also, a woman having her first baby when she's only in her thirties is still referred to medically as an "elderly primipara," meaning old first-time mom! Statistically, she's more likely to have problems, which is why doctors classify her that way. (Some doctors now say "mature primipara," which is at least a little less jarring!)

Now you know why one of life's greatest ironies is that you may faithfully use birth control for many years only to discover that when you finally test the equipment, you don't get pregnant. As month after month slips by and your period keeps coming, you may start to panic. Is it him? Is it you? Words such as "infertile, "barren," and "sterile" can haunt you. Just seeing someone else cuddling her baby tends to bring on the tears. Standard advice is that if you're under thirty-five, you should try for a year before seeing a specialist. If you're over thirty-five, the rule is to give it six months. Plenty of people don't wait that long, though, and I think that's wise. Certainly, both of you should have a complete physical. Plenty of health issues can contribute to infertility and many of them are correctable. Especially if the infamous biological clock is ticking, why waste time?

Here's a perfect example. A woman who was not one of my regular patients came to me for help after years of trying to get pregnant. By then she was in her mid-thirties. She had been to several fertility specialists but had never received a diagnosis. Her husband's sperm count and motility were normal. I wish she had known what you learned in chapter 3 of this book about collecting your own health records! She walked into my office with no paper trail in hand at all so I had to rely entirely on the history she could remember. Listening to her, something told me that a simple, easily treatable cause for her inability to conceive had somehow been overlooked. I palpated her thyroid glands on either side of her neck with my fingers. The glands felt "full" or slightly swollen. Then I ordered complete blood work including an especially sensitive test for thyroid problems that isn't always done. Her results came back with the highest score for thyroid-stimulating hormone (TSH) I had ever seen. It was close to 100, although the norm is less than 5! This tipped me off to the fact that she was making almost no thyroid at all. The TSH sends a signal when the body should make more thyroid. In her case the TSH wasn't getting any results so it just kept sending

What Are My Options as a Woman with a Female Partner?

Many female couples in committed relationships choose to have children. One option is to use Assisted Reproductive Technology (ART) (see page 160) to get pregnant with donor sperm from a sperm bank. Some women use sperm from male friends, either heterosexual or homosexual. If you're over thirty-five, you may want or need to use both donor eggs and donor sperm. Some partners decide that only one of them will get pregnant and others decide that both of them will. Of course, you could also adopt. Whatever the case, be sure that each partner has legal paperwork that allows her to seek medical care for your child or children. Laws vary from state to state. All of this can be complicated and costly for you, but the bottom line is that you can be a mother just like any other woman if that's want you want.

louder and louder messages to no avail. Low thyroid or hypothyroidism can be a cause of infertility since the hormones in a woman's body work in concert. I started her on thyroid therapy right away.

Because of her insurance, she went back to her original doctor and I didn't hear from her again. Then by chance several years later I ran into her at a community event. She had a three-year-old, a toddler, and she was pregnant again! When she saw me she blushed and apologized for not getting in touch to thank me. "I meant to call you," she said, "but I've been really busy!" I once had three in diapers at the same time so I could relate!

As my story about the patient with hypothyroidism shows, infertility isn't always intractable, although it sometimes is. Some common causes are chlamydia and gonorrhea (see chapter 2), and endometriosis, fibroids, and PCOS (see chapter 7). In addition, in January of 2009 researchers at the UCLA School of Public Health found the first evidence that perfluorinated chemicals (PFCs) that are commonly used in food packaging, pesticides, clothing, upholstery, carpets, and personal care products may be associated with infertility in women. Beyond that, you or your partner may have structural abnormalities of your reproductive organs or various hormonal imbalances. After you've had your complete physicals, the next step is to consult one or more fertility specialists. Years ago, before the advent of Assisted Reproductive Technology (ART) with the birth in 1978 of the first "test tube baby," you would have had limited treatment options. Today you have an impressive range of choices. However, keep in mind that ART is no clambake. Be sure you are fully informed about the costs both fiscal and physical and keep in mind that results are far from guaranteed. I don't want to discourage you from doing everything you can to have a baby if that's a dream you're not willing to dismiss easily. All I'm saying is that I hope you'll go into this with your eyes wide open.

I'm thinking about a dear friend who had endometriosis. For her, the ART experience was fraught with roller-coaster emotions, pain, huge medical bills, and in the end, failure. First she was put into drug-induced artificial menopause, complete with mood swings and hot flashes, to shrink the runaway endometrial implants that were growing where they shouldn't be. Then she was pumped full of mega doses of hormones to stimulate her egg production. Next came the painful procedure for "harvesting" the eggs. They were fertilized with her husband's sperm and the resulting embryos were inserted into her uterus—another procedure she does not remember with any fondness—in hopes that one or more would implant. That didn't happen even though she tried three times. At that point she decided that her body had been assaulted enough. She went on to adopt a beautiful daughter from China whom she and her husband love with all their hearts. "Looking back, I honestly wish I had never tried IVF," she told me. "But I'm actually glad I turned out to be infertile. Otherwise we would never have met Lian. I can't imagine life without her."

Certainly there are also many ART stories with very happy endings. I hope that if you try ART, your story will be added to that pantheon. You know that I wish you well! Even so, I wouldn't be true to my mission if I didn't give you the whole truth so that you can make informed decisions about how to proceed if pregnancy eludes you.

Best case scenario, of course, would be if you stopped using birth control, hopped into bed, and conceived then and there—or at least shortly thereafter. It happens! But whether you get pregnant the old-fashioned way or with the help of some form of ART, your body is on automatic pilot once you've conceived. With no conscious effort on your part, it will simply go about its business and begin to turn a ball of cells into a fetus that will, if all goes well, emerge from your womb as a full-fledged human being. That qualifies as nothing short of a miracle in my opinion!

GREAT WITH CHILD: PREGNANCY AND CHILDBIRTH

A big difference in your experience as a pregnant woman compared to your mother's, or even perhaps your older sister's, is that more prenatal genetic tests are now available. Another fairly recent development is evidence of how certain foods and substances can affect the fetus. Finally, you have more choices than ever before when it comes to making your "birth plan." Let's go over each of those topics one at a time

PRENATAL DIAGNOSTIC PROCEDURES AND TESTS

When I was pregnant with my first child, having an ultrasound to find out the sex of the fetus had just come into vogue. I was adamantly opposed to that. Maybe I'm superstitious but I just didn't want Mother Nature to be upset by my fooling with her! However, I was assured by many of the wise older women who worked with me that because I was carrying my pregnancy entirely in the front, as though I had swallowed a beach ball, this meant I was going to have a boy. I kind of went with that, but using technology rather than relying on old wives' tales somehow didn't seem right. I've heard young women today say the same thing, although just about everybody does opt to find out whether to paint the nursery pink or blue. I'm actually still glad I waited for the surprise. I remember the moment my son popped out. The nurses knew our names were either Sarah or Zachary and they immediately cried, "It's a Zachary!" Their joyful proclamation has never left me.

Of course, the more important reason for having an ultrasound is to make sure the baby is developing normally, and I did do that. I just told the doctor to keep the sex secret. Fortunately for me, the fetus showed no signs of any problems. I was never put in the position of considering my options if there seemed to be trouble ahead. Now that prenatal screening and procedures are common, especially for women over thirty-five, I think you and your partner need to have a frank discussion about why you do or don't want information about possible birth defects and what you would do if the news was not good. This is especially true if conditions such as cystic fibrosis, Tay-Sachs, or spina bifida run in your family. It's equally true if you are over thirty-five and therefore at increased risk of having a Down syndrome baby.

Sarah Palin, the 2008 Republican candidate for vice president, said that she had the potentially risky invasive procedure called amniocentesis (see page 163) only because she wanted to be forewarned about whether or not she was carrying a Down syndrome fetus. Since the risk of miscarriage from the procedure is as great as the risk of having a Down syndrome child when the maternal age is over thirty-five, that logic escapes me. If you're going to continue the pregnancy no matter what, how have you gained anything by taking a chance that you'll miscarry as a result of amniocentesis?

True, while you're still pregnant you could do some research about what caring for a special needs child will mean for you and your family. However, beyond that, the advance notice doesn't seem to me to be worth the risk if you really mean it when you say you want the baby regardless of what the test results tell you. Also, I have a friend who lost a perfectly healthy baby because of amniocentesis. As always, don't let anyone pressure you into opting for a procedure just because it's available. Only you, and your partner, if you have one, can decide what's right for you.

Screening Procedures

If you're under thirty-five and have no family history of birth defects, meaning relatives born with genetic abnormalities, the only tests you'll probably need are blood tests and ultrasound. The upside of these tests is that there's no risk of harming you or the fetus. The downside is that the results are not definitive. What you'll learn regarding whether or not you'll give birth to a baby with what we commonly call "birth defects" is the odds of that happening. If either of the screening procedures points to the possibility of fetal abnormalities, you may be given the option of further testing.

Diagnostic Procedures

Amniocentesis

This test is offered to women thirty-five and over and it's done at about sixteen weeks. The doctor will insert a needle into your abdomen and draw out amniotic fluid. The diagnosis of Down syndrome (trisomy 13) and cystic fibrosis is definitive. There is, as I said earlier, a risk of miscarriage.

Chorionic Villus Sampling

This is a newer test offered to women over thirty-five and done at about ten to twelve weeks. Like amniocentesis, it carries the risk of miscarriage. The doctor will either insert a needle into your abdomen or a catheter into your cervix. The advantage of this test over amniocentesis is that if you plan to terminate the pregnancy should the fetus turn out to have abnormalities, you can do so earlier and therefore more safely.

WHAT TO AVOID WHEN YOU'RE PREGNANT

Remember that you'll be two weeks along before you miss your period. During that time, the zygote will already have morphed into a multi-celled blastocyst that traveled down your fallopian tube and burrowed into the lining of your uterus to start receiving nourishment. If you're trying to get pregnant, begin taking prenatal vitamins with folic acid right away and also make lifestyle changes now rather than after the test strip tells you you've conceived!

- Quit smoking. I know, I know. Quitting is really tough. But please get support and do this for yourself and your baby!
- Stop drinking alcohol. Some guidelines say that an occasional drink is okay but most research shows that any alcohol intake may adversely affect the fetus. I strongly advise you to give up alcohol altogether for the duration. True, your mom may have had a drink every now and then when she was pregnant and

What Causes Miscarriages?

Most miscarriages are nature's way of eliminating a mistake. Usually the fetus had a chromosomal abnormality. However, women who experience two or more miscarriages may have an auto-immune disorder or perhaps fibroids that are competing with the fetus for blood supply. Be sure to go for testing if you have repeated miscarriages. Also, recognize that almost all women who miscarry experience real grief over the loss. Yet because miscarriages typically occur during the first trimester, probably only your partner and close family and friends will even know. Putting a brave face on in public can be difficult but you don't have to go it alone. You can find comfort, solace, and hope in support groups both actual and virtual.

you turned out fine. Still, she was pregnant before the risks were known. Now that you have the information she didn't have, why not do everything you can to ensure that your baby won't be harmed?

- Talk to your doctor about prescription and over-the-counter medications. Many of them are not safe to take during pregnancy.

- Cut out caffeine. Here again, your mom probably did drink coffee during her pregnancies. But as she used to tell you when you were little, two wrongs don't make a right! According to a 2008 study published in the *American Journal of Obstetrics and Gynecology*, caffeine doubles the risk of miscarriage. Remember that not only coffee but also tea, colas, energy drinks, and some other soft drinks contain caffeine. Even if you make it past the time when most miscarriages occur, caffeine could up your risk of preterm labor. Tapering off caffeine will help prevent withdrawal symptoms such as headaches and jitteriness but if you decide to quit cold turkey, rest assured that you'll feel fine again in a few days!

YOUR BIRTH PLAN

The practice of writing a birth plan that lets health-care providers in on your ideal scenario for the birthing process is fairly new. However, it has its origins in the early 1970s pendulum swing away from routinely medicalized births and back toward so-called "natural childbirth." Scores of women read *Thank You, Dr. Lamaze* and went to classes to learn the breathing techniques that might help them avoid anesthesia or drugs during labor. Husbands went along so that they could be labor coaches in the delivery room instead of pacing outside in the waiting room. The goal was for the woman to remain "awake and aware" and for the husband to be present at the creation. All of that has an obvious appeal and it not only plays into Everywoman's desire to be the Earth Mother who delivers with relative ease, but it also promises, correctly, that the baby won't be at risk from medication given to the mother. In the wake of that development, midwives came back into favor and such practices as home births and laboring in a hot tub got a lot of media attention.

However, what wasn't mentioned back then was the fact that in the centuries before modern medicine came into full flower, "natural" childbirth often meant that neither the mother nor the baby survived. Yet the use of the word "natural" often had the effect of laying a guilt trip on women who didn't "succeed" in having a vaginal birth without medication. Worse yet, women who "failed" to give birth vaginally and ended up with an emergency C-section really beat themselves up. (Incidentally, the phrase "cesarean section" does not derive from Julius Caesar, as was erroneously reported for years in no less a source than the *Oxford English Dictionary*. The etymology is most likely from the Greek word "caedere," meaning "to cut." However, this surgery was well-known in Caesar's day, so the practice of intervening to save the mother and baby when "natural" childbirth isn't going well is nothing new!)

Happily, in the decades since the 1970s, the stance on natural childbirth has softened considerably. Most women and their partners still attend childbirth education classes, but the mothers-to-be feel less pressure now to "succeed." Also, many women elect to have labor induced or even elect to have a C-section. A 2002 article in the *British Medical Journal* reported on the high rate of elective C-sections among upper-class women around the world, but particularly in Brazil. One of the reasons cited for this choice by the Brazilian women was that they'd have less pain with sex after the birth. (Those rascals! They also invented the Brazilian waxing of pubic hair.)

At this point, you have a range of choices to consider when you sit down to write your Birth Plan. Keep in mind, though, that this is one time in your life when the "best-laid plans . . . often go awry," to quote the poet Robert Burns. I talk a lot about taking charge of your own health care, and I do want you to be at the center of your birthing experience. However, I hope you won't set the bar too high or be disappointed if things don't turn out the way you had envisioned. Here's a partial list of what could happen in spite of your birth plan:

- You might have preterm labor and need to forego the midwife in order to get to a hospital where a premature baby can be cared for in the neonatal intensive-care unit.
- You might have precipitate labor that goes so fast you make headlines in the local paper because your husband had to pull over on the way to the hospital and deliver the baby himself in the car.
- You might have "inefficient" labor, also called dystocia, and find that after many hours you're still not dilated and need a C-section to get the baby out before the placenta stops nourishing him.
- You might not go into labor at all and need an induction or a C-section because your baby is postmature and therefore not getting nutrients.
- Or, in the best of all possible worlds, you could go into labor right on your due date, manage just fine with breathing techniques, and pop out your precious bundle with not much trouble at all.

In other words, anything can happen! All that matters in the end is that you and the baby—or babies—are alive and well. This is not a contest. No woman's way of delivering is superior to yours.

I know that can be a difficult concept to grasp if you've always been a high achiever and a hard worker, but we're not dealing here with an outcome you can control. Your body is in command. All you can do is to learn about your options and then be grateful for medical intervention if you and the baby need it.

OH, BABY! YOUR BODY, YOUR EMOTIONS, AND YOUR LIFE AS A MOM

After the baby is born, life will never be the same again. You knew that going in, but only in the abstract. Once you've delivered and you're home safe, the round-the-clock reality of mothering a newborn can be all but overwhelming. Maybe you're also recuperating from a cesarean or from the stitches you needed after you gave birth vaginally. Maybe, as I did after my first son was born, you're dealing with a very painful hemorrhoid and some stress incontinence. Perhaps you're also having other vaginal, bowel, or urinary tract problems. You're probably also frustrated because you still can't fit back into your regular clothes. Check out chapters 7, 8, 9, and 11 for help and reassurance on all of these concerns. You'll get through this! In fact, as I've pointed out elsewhere, my postpartum bowel episode actually prompted me to make lifestyle changes that have done my overall health a lot of good to this day.

Of course, beyond the issues you may be dealing with "down there," you could also be having trouble nursing. You've heard time and again that you should give your baby the benefits of breast milk, but please don't let the purists make you feel as though you're flunking Motherhood 101. Go ahead and get help from a trained lactation consultant if you want to, and pump if that seems to be what's called for, but resist letting yourself feel as though you're in competition with the La Leche League leader who's successfully suckling her little bundle next to you on the park bench. Remember also that even though "breast milk is the best milk," generations of formula-fed babies have grown up to be healthy and happy adults. I'm not saying you shouldn't give breastfeeding your best shot, but if you do end up reaching for the formula, you're not a horrible person.

I supplemented my breast milk with some bottle feedings for my firstborn as well as my twins. Trust me, my three strapping grown sons are proof positive that what really matters is that your baby gets enough to eat. Just as important, you need some shut-eye! Most women are surprised to learn that breastfeeding causes a woman's body to enter a state of virtual menopause, complete with plummeting hormones that may cause mood swings and trouble with sexual desire. Add sleep deprivation to the mix, along with being sore in one or more spots below the belt, and you have a surefire recipe for the baby blues! I don't want to make light of postpartum depression because it's a real and severe disorder that requires treatment. But only about 10 percent of new mothers suffer from it. The rest of us are simply worn down from hormonal changes, the baby's demands, and the aftereffects of pregnancy and childbirth. I remember crying even though I knew I was blessed. My emotions were all over the place. Having sex hurt and I had dreams of the baby being one big mouth while I was just an extension of him! If you go through anything similar, know that you're not alone. My advice is to do something, anything, that will make you feel that you still matter beyond being a vessel for milk production and a twenty-four/seven first responder to your baby's needs. Also, consider getting some help, at least during the early weeks. Maybe your mother or mother-in-law can pitch in, or perhaps your partner can get a few weeks of family leave. Another option if you can afford it is to hire a baby nurse or a "doula" who is trained to support you through the birth process and during your adjustment to motherhood.

Even an hour to yourself when you can read a trashy novel or get a manicure or call a coworker to catch up on the gossip back at the office can work wonders. The baby will benefit, too. The better you feel both physically and emotionally, the more you'll be able to give her the love and attention she needs. Someday soon, the first crazy weeks will be nothing but a blurry memory and you'll be happily playing peek-a-boo with the best little baby in the world!

That completes my advice for your journey through the fertile years. Whether you choose to have children or not, you'll be dealing with birth control for many years to come. If you do have one or more children, you'll also be busy bringing up the baby or the brood. Not only that, but for many of us this season of our lives includes working outside the home, maintaining a good marital relationship, and maybe at some point coping as a suddenly single mother. Plenty of "sandwich generation" women also care for aging parents. Hang in there! A new season is coming, one that has gotten a bad rap but that is in fact full of sweet surprises. My next mission is to give you advice and encouragement about how to make the most of menopause and the bonus years beyond it. Go ahead and take a sneak peek even if you're not nearing this milestone just yet!

6

The Bonus Years

Making the Most of Menopause and Beyond

The average life expectancy of a woman born in 1900 was forty-nine. Since the age when most women have their final period is about fifty-two, she might not have reached that milestone. You, on the other hand, are statistically likely to be around to enjoy a substantial number of years when birth control is no longer necessary, the nest is empty, and retirement or an "encore career" has made the rat race a mere memory. In addition, the low-maintenance pleasures of grandparenting may be yours. And if you're lucky enough to be among the estimated 20 percent of women who experience few or no menopausal symptoms, you may sail through this life event wondering what all the fuss is about when it comes to the debate over the various types of Hormone Therapy including bio-identical hormones. Still, no less a source than the National Institutes of Health reports that some 60 percent of women have symptoms bothersome enough to merit treatment. What's more, an additional 20 percent have symptoms that are severe and even disabling. In other words, menopause is no picnic for a great many women. I speak from experience! Also, even women who have an easy time of it need to learn to live well with the new reality of a postmenopausal body.

Lost in the chorus of conflicting claims about what women should or shouldn't do for symptomatic relief of menopausal symptoms is the fact that menopause ushers in lasting transformations in a woman's body. In other words, menopause really is a "change." After you have had your final period ever and the hot flashes— if any—simmer down at last, you are different in six important ways. Some of these are attributable solely to menopause while others also have to do with the effects of aging in general. Together they constitute that "new reality" I mentioned and they all need your attention if you're going to maintain your health.

Here is what will be new about your postmenopausal body.

1. The risk of heart disease increases. As estrogen levels decrease, we lose our edge over men when it comes to warding off cardiac problems and strokes.

2. Belly fat increases. Our fat distribution shifts from the protective "pear-shaped" zone around the hips and thighs to the more dangerous "apple-shaped" zone of belly fat typical of men. This puts us at higher risk for metabolic syndrome, type 2 diabetes, and the cascade of conditions this disease can engender.

3. Blood pressure goes up. Even women who have always had low blood pressure and who are not overweight or sedentary can experience an increase that puts the BP higher than the recommended 130/80.

4. Metabolism slows down, but mostly this happens if you slow down and lose fat-burning muscle mass.

5. Bone density decreases. Virtually all postmenopausal women eventually have a condition called osteopenia. The risk of fractures goes up and if osteoporosis develops, the risk of fractures goes up further still.

6. Vulvar tissues atrophy. All menopausal women experience a thinning of the tissues of the vulva including the vagina, urethra, and the labia that can lead to problems. Almost half develop a more advanced version commonly called atrophic vaginitis (discussed later in this chapter).

I, for one, find facing up to these realities of the postmenopausal body to be empowering rather than depressing. Knowing the truth about how we have changed inside gives us the opportunity to take preventive measures that will keep us well.

You won't be surprised to hear that I'm going to hit home once again my message about making wise lifestyle choices. In addition though, as

What Are the Definitions of "Perimenopause," "Menopause," and "Postmenopause"?

The term "perimenopause" first appeared in the Merriam Webster dictionary in 1962. The literal meaning is "around the menopause." Perimenopause refers not only to the years when ovulation has started to shut down, usually during the mid-forties, but also to the twelve months after the last period ever. This is because cessation of the menses can only be diagnosed retroactively.

All the years after perimenopause are called postmenopause although symptoms may persist. Technically, the word "menopause"—and it's not a pause at all but a full stop!—refers only to the last menstrual cycle. Remember, you won't know for sure that it was the final one until twelve months have passed with no periods. However, in popular parlance "menopause" is most often used to refer to the whole process. For example, people say, "She's going through menopause." Even doctors often refer to "menopausal patients."

you'll learn later in this chapter, my Five Factors for Selecting a Hormone Therapy Option can also help you as long as you are not on my list of those for whom HT is not a good option. Incidentally, HT is sometimes called hormone replacement therapy (HRT) or menopause hormone therapy (MHT). The terms are interchangeable.

Because I'm a doctor of internal medicine who treats the whole patient rather than a gynecologist who focuses on the reproductive system, my mission is to make you aware of how menopause and aging affect your entire system. A lot of us tackle the external markers of aging by coloring our hair, using "age-defying" or "rejuvenating" skincare products, or perhaps opting for plastic surgery. That's fine if those surface upgrades make you feel good about yourself. But how much better it is to team them with smart strategies to combat the effects of the internal transformations of the third age of our lives! I'll detail those strategies for you including a safe, effective, and protective HT regimen with FDA-approved bio-identical hormones. I use it myself. First, though, I want you to understand exactly what goes on as you progress through perimenopause.

WHAT HAPPENS DURING "THE CHANGE"

In the 1970s when menopause was still a taboo topic, the groundbreaking television show *All in the Family* aired a now-classic scene in which Archie Bunker, a lovable working-class bigot, loses patience when his wife has a hot flash while eating soup:

> **Archie Bunker:** *I know all about your woman's troubles there, Edith, but when I had the hernia that time, I didn't make you wear the truss. If you're gonna have the change of life, you gotta do it right now. I'm gonna give you just thirty seconds. Now c'mon and change.*

Edith Bunker: *Can I finish my soup first?*

If only menopause were so simple! Unfortunately, we don't have an inner switch that would turn off female fertility with one flick. Instead, the process is a gradual one during which the ovaries produce less and less estrogen, progesterone, and testosterone. Your adrenal glands do go on making a certain amount of testosterone and other hormones, some

Will I Go into Menopause If I Have a Hysterectomy?

That depends. If you have the kind of surgery that leaves your ovaries intact, they will shut down their hormone production gradually just as they would have if you still had a uterus. The process may be a little faster than it would have been. You obviously won't have periods and you won't be able to get pregnant. Otherwise, you'll experience perimenopause in pretty much the same way as anybody else might.

If you have your ovaries removed, however, you'll go into instant and complete "surgical menopause." The symptoms, including frequent hot flashes, are predictably severe. I recommend having a transdermal HT patch applied before you're wheeled into the OR unless hormones are contraindicated. (See page 183 for a discussion of contraindications.) That way when your endogenous (internal) hormone levels suddenly plummet, you'll have exogenous (from the outside) hormones already circulating in your bloodstream. What I really recommend, though, is that you avoid an oophorectomy—the removal of your ovaries—if at all possible. After your eggs are gone, your ovaries continue to make hormones vital to your well-being, although in lesser amounts than when you were fertile. (See chapter 7, page 231 for more information.)

Can I Get Pregnant after Menopause with Donor Eggs?

Yes, you could use Assisted Reproductive Technology and receive donor eggs. Headlines have been made around the world as women well past childbearing age have given birth, including a sixty-seven-year-old retired university professor in Romania and a fifty-five-year-old woman in Michigan who was the surrogate for her own triplet granddaughters. The stuff of science fiction is now a reality, but the expense and risk of the procedures that make late-in-life pregnancies possible are huge. Also, while the Michigan triplets do have a young mother with a good chance of nurturing them to adulthood, the child of the Romanian woman will be lucky if she has Mom around to celebrate with her on her thirteenth birthday. I, for one, take a dim view of artificially created postmenopausal pregnancies. Still, the option is there. Of course, the flip side of this is that the donor eggs come from young women who have elected to undertake a lengthy and painful procedure in order to sell their eggs. If you're still fertile and you're considering doing this, please be very well informed before making your decision.

of which are then changed to estrogen in your fat cells—especially belly or "visceral" fat cells. However, this estrogen is not as potent as what you once had. All of these hormonal changes work together to precipitate a disruption of your previously regular cycle of ovulation so that your periods become unpredictable and often heavy. Over time, about ten years for most of us, any eggs and follicles that are still left in the ovaries degenerate. When the last available egg ripens and travels down one of your fallopian tubes, you have your final period. As I said, the last period usually happens at the age of fifty-two although smokers typically go through menopause several years earlier than that. Keep in mind, though, that you won't know you're no longer fertile until a full year has gone by with no periods, so do continue using birth control—and condoms even after that to protect against STIs if you have new partners.

Also, if you're taking birth control pills (see sidebar on birth control pills on page 189) or cyclic HT, you won't know when your egg production stops because you'll continue to experience "withdrawal bleeds" every month. However, the bleeds from HT will eventually lighten and may disappear altogether, especially if you're at a healthy weight and don't have excess belly fat. Still, you may want to get a blood test to confirm that you've gone through menopause and can safely stop using contraceptives. You will need to stop your hormones for five days or more before getting this simple blood test that will show that you are producing a very high level of follicle-stimulating hormone (FSH). Back in chapter 4, you learned that FSH kicks in at puberty to cause the follicles to mature and the eggs to ripen. At menopause after all the eggs are gone, FSH starts sending stronger and stronger signals. You might think of this as though the FSH is frustrated because there's no response! The high level of FSH is normal and it's not harmful at all.

By now menopause is no longer shrouded in secrecy and women who would never have discussed their periods in polite company wisecrack about their hot flashes anywhere from the office to cocktail parties. However, all the empowering bravado about "red-hot mamas" aside, the infamous symptoms can be truly disabling for plenty of women. You probably already know about the hallmark complaints. Along with hot flashes, women experience erratic periods, sleep disturbances, night sweats, memory lapses, and mood swings. Some women also have heart palpitations, "pins and needles" or "crawly" skin, joint pain, headaches, and breast tenderness. Another postmenopausal symptom is facial hair that sprouts when estrogen levels drop and androgens predominate. My postmenopausal sister-in-law was only half joking when she told her daughters to pluck out her chin hairs if she's ever too frail or demented to do it herself!

Reduced libido can also happen. However, the reason you're not in the mood may have more to do with physical issues such as a dry vagina and the thinning skin of your labia than with an actual lack of desire. Sex during menopause is such an important topic that I've devoted a whole section of this chapter to it. (Okay, skip ahead if you can't wait, but promise me you'll come back and read all of the other life-enhancing information I have for you as well!)

HORMONE THERAPY (HT): BOON OR BANE?

As you know by now, I am against thinking of any medication as a magic bullet that gets you out of the need to take what I call the "Life-style Pill." Later in this chapter I'll go over what you can do not only for symptomatic relief during menopause but also for a lifetime of good health in your new postmenopausal body. However, as a physician and as a woman myself, I strongly believe that there is also a place for safe and effective hormone therapy in the lives of vast numbers of women. I've already discussed testosterone therapy for low libido in chapter 2. Now I'm going to explain estrogen and progesterone therapy for menopausal symptoms and as protection against certain health problems. I know that you may well be confused about whether or not HT is a good option for you. HT's history has always been fraught with controversy.

To clarify the salient issues for you in the most succinct manner possible, I'm going to present them first as a list. After you've studied the bullet points and absorbed a basic understanding of this complex and often confusing topic, you can go on to read my in-depth explanation that follows the list.

- **What are conjugated estrogens?** *Conjugated* in this context means "formed by the union of two compounds." The phrase *conjugated estrogens* refers to an FDA-approved synthetic product derived from the urine of pregnant mares—hence the brand name "Premarin." It also refers to an FDA-approved plant-based product called Cenestin. The molecular structure of these products is not identical to the estrogen produced by a woman's body. No one knows whether or not this is clinically significant.

- **What is unopposed estrogen?** This phrase refers to estrogen that is not balanced by progesterone. In the 1970s, researchers linked unopposed estrogen therapy with an increased risk of uterine cancer.

- **What are bio-identical hormones?** These are products with molecular structures that are the same as those of the hormones produced by a woman's body before menopause. Again, no one knows whether or not this is clinically significant. Bio-identical hormones are often called "natural." However, they are synthesized in laboratories from plant sources such as Mexican wild yams (not the same as sweet potatoes!) and soy. In that sense, they can be called "synthetic."

- **Are there any bio-identical hormones approved by the FDA?** Yes. Several bio-identical estrogen (estradiol) products made from yams were approved during the 1990s. One, with the brand name Estrace, is made from both yams and soy. An FDA-approved progesterone product, Prometrium, is a "micronized" form of the hormone that is easy for the body to process.

- **What is a compounding pharmacy?** These are pharmacies that custom mix drugs according to a physician's prescription. Media attention has recently focused on their role in creating bio-identical preparations. One reason a doctor might tailor a prescription for a menopausal woman would be to treat her with testosterone for low libido. Some doctors customize an HT prescription based on the results of a saliva test but these tests are unreliable. Also, the position of the American College of Obstetricians and Gynecologists on this issue is that "hormone therapy does not require customized dosing."

- **Why doesn't the FDA approve preparations made by compounding pharmacists?** The FDA can only approve products that are standardized and that have been shown in clinical trials to be safe and effective. A corollary of this fact is that insurance companies may not pay for hormones compounded by a pharmacy. Therefore the cost to the consumer can be greater than for pharmaceutical-grade hormones.

- **Can herbal supplements relieve menopausal symptoms?** Probably not and they may not be safe. A 2005 study done by the National Center for Complementary and Alternative Medicine (NCCAM) of the National Institutes of Health (NIH), reported that there is not as yet enough evidence to support the belief that "botanicals" such as black cohosh, red clover, ginseng, dong quai, and kava reduce menopausal symptoms or that they cause no harm. None of these preparations are FDA-approved. NCCAM also cautions that herbal remedies can have adverse interactions with over-the-counter and prescription medications.

- **What does "oral medication" mean?** This refers to drugs in pill or capsule form. Among the drawbacks of oral hormone medications is that when the liver processes them, they stimulate proteins associated with heart disease and stroke.

- **What does "transdermal medication" mean?** This refers to products such as patches, creams, and gels, which allow drugs to be absorbed through the skin. This method bypasses the liver. Another way to bypass the liver is to deliver medication through the vagina such as with intravaginal estrogen.

- **What is "continuous therapy"?** This means that estrogen and progesterone therapy are taken every day without interruption even though a pre-menopausal woman does not produce progesterone every day of the month. A combination pill such as Prempro (Premarin plus Provera, a synthetic version of progesterone called progestin) constitutes continuous therapy.

Women may bleed erratically at first but most women stop
bleeding altogether on continuous therapy.

- **What is cyclical therapy?** This means that a form of continuous
  estrogen therapy is teamed with separate progesterone therapy
  that is purposely interrupted for several days a month to mimic
  a woman's natural hormonal cycle. Women will typically bleed
  in a cyclic fashion, although the bleeding is usually minimal and
  sometimes stops altogether.

- **If a woman is going to use an HT regimen, when should
  she start?** The earlier during perimenopause the better. HT
  should not be started by post-menopausal women in the hopes
  of preventing health problems such as Alzheimer's or heart
  disease. There is no evidence that HT provides this kind of
  protection and starting hormones that late may pose health
  risks.

- **Why are current HT doses lower than in the past?** Low doses
  have been shown to be effective and they are safer than the
  higher doses prescribed in previous years.

- **Does HT significantly increase the risk of breast cancer?**
  The risk is small, especially when it comes to women who
  don't have high risk factors in the first place. (See the sidebar
  "Who Shouldn't Take Hormone Therapy?" on page 183.)
  Women who have disabling symptoms of menopause may
  decide in conjunction with their physicians that the benefits of
  HT outweigh the slight risk. Also, the risk has been shown to
  disappear completely within a short time if a woman stops HT.

- **How long should a woman stay on an HT regimen?** The
  answer varies from woman to woman. Many women stop after
  symptoms such as hot flashes and night sweats have subsided.
  Other women who continue to be bothered by symptoms such as
  vaginal dryness and itching that compromise sexual pleasure may
  choose in conjunction with their physicians to continue a safe

and effective form of HT indefinitely. (See my Five Factors on page 185 for the regimen I recommend.)

Now that you have a good grasp of what's involved in considering HT, let's look closely at the timeline of events precipitated by the latest highly publicized scare. In 2002 the National Institutes of Health abruptly halted the Women's Health Initiative (WHI) study because the risks of Premarin and Prempro were proving to be greater than the benefits. Headlines that were splashed across newspapers as well as articles that were rushed into the major women's magazines warned that HT had been shown to raise the risk of heart disease and breast cancer. The study also showed that the risks of bone fractures and colon cancers were reduced, but that did little to assuage everyone's fears. Scores of women immediately stopped their HT regimens.

I was one of them. However, I wasn't willing to give up on HT altogether. For one thing, because I had read the fine print of the WHI study, I knew that it was flawed. This has been confirmed in the years since. The subjects were not perimenopausal women seeking symptomatic relief. The participants in the trial, with the goal of finding out whether HT could protect women against heart disease, were largely postmenopausal women. The mean age was sixty-three. Most of them were overweight or obese and most of them had not taken HT when they were younger or they had stopped years earlier. Not only that, but most of them had no symptoms or only mild symptoms. After all, why would a woman with disabling symptoms agree to be in a trial in which she might be one of those receiving a placebo? Also, the researchers were discouraged from enrolling women with severe hot flashes and other symptoms because the active treatment would markedly relieve symptoms and this would essentially "unblind" the researchers because they would then know which pill the symptomatic patients were taking. Those facts said to me that the results of the study were far from representative of the effects of HT on women like me. I had started

Who Shouldn't Take Hormone Therapy?

Your own doctor will go over all the aspects of your medical history with you so that you can make a personal decision. However, in general HT is contraindicated if:

- you smoke;
- you are significantly overweight or obese and therefore making excess endogenous (internal) estrogen in your fat cells even though you are no longer making enough progesterone to balance it out;
- you are a breast cancer survivor;
- you have a strong family history of breast cancer;
- you are postmenopausal in your late fifties or older and you have never taken HT or you stopped years earlier. Starting now may pose a slightly increased risk of heart disease in the first year of use, and breast cancer with long-term use. However, you may be a candidate for intravaginal estrogen to relieve the symptoms of atrophic vaginitis (see page 193).

therapy early when the timing was right and I didn't have breast cancer as a family risk factor so that wasn't a worry. On the flip side, I did have concerns about cardiac disease and low bone density so I wanted the possible protection that hormome therapy could give me.

FDA-APPROVED BIO-IDENTICALS

Even so, because I had been taking a combination of synthetic oral estrogen and progestin, I did reconsider my HT options. In fact I wrote an op-ed piece that was published in the *Philadelphia Inquirer* explaining why I chose my new regimen. First, I switched to Vivelle-dot, a transdermal ("through the skin") patch that had been approved by the FDA

What Are My Choices for a Patch?

I use the Vivelle patch but there are several other brands. They all work equally well. Vivelle comes in a variety of doses. The 0.05 dose of estrogen acts in a manner similar to the most popular oral dose of Premarin at 0.625mg. However, many women can gradually shift to even lower estrogen doses from the patch, such as the 0.025 mg patch. With lower estrogen, less oral Prometrium (the micronized progesterone) will be needed because the uterine lining will be less likely to build up.

in 1994. It delivers a bio-identical form of estradiol (a type of estrogen) derived from yams. The molecular structure is chemically the same as the estradiol produced by a woman's body before menopause.

Next, because the dangers of taking estrogen that is unopposed by progesterone have long been known, I coupled the patch with cyclical oral doses of Prometrium, a bio-identical micronized form of progesterone that had been approved by the FDA in 1998. Again, the source of the hormone is yams and the molecular structure is the same as that of endogenous progesterone. There is to date no transdermal FDA-approved form of progesterone. If there were, I would prefer it to the oral medication. (Prometrium isn't used in birth control pills. See chapter 5.)

The patch delivers a very low dose of estrogen that goes directly into the bloodstream rather than going to the liver as all orally ingested pills do. The liver is nature's digestive clearinghouse. When you take hormones orally, you need a dose that's about ten times higher than the dose required if you have a patch because the liver will break down the dose and send only about one-tenth of it into your system to do its work on most tissues in the body.

Beyond that, any estrogen delivered transdermally—whether by the patch, the spray recently approved by the FDA, or a cream or gel—doesn't

Dr. Marie's Five Factors
for Selecting an HT Option

I based my personal regimen on the following factors that I find most important for a safe and effective HT that can not only offer symptomatic relief but also protection for the postmenopausal body.

1. **Timing.** The sooner you begin HT during perimenopause, the better. The timing of hormones is key for optimizing the benefits to the heart, the bones, and also for cognitive function. Conversely, hormones started late in life are not good for the heart and brain.

2. **Delivery.** Opt for a transdermal method rather than sending the hormones to your liver by swallowing a pill.

3. **Low dosage.** The higher the dose of estrogen, the greater the risks.

4. **Periodic or "cyclic" progesterone.** Avoid synthetic progestin such as Provera and regimens that keep you on progesterone continuously. These increase health risks.

5. **Duration.** Even after menopausal symptoms have subsided, this regimen can be beneficial lifelong for many women by making the vagina plump and moist again and cutting the risk of osteoporosis, colon cancer, and heart disease. These benefits may or may not outweigh the slightly increased risk of breast cancer after four, five, or more years of use for any given woman. Each woman and her physician need to make an individual decision about whether or not to continue.

carry the risk of an increased tendency to blood clots or high blood pressure. In addition, it doesn't cause an increase in blood inflammation as measured by a simple, inexpensive blood test called the C-reactive protein test. It does help to improve blood cholesterol although the "good cholesterol" will not go up as high as it does with oral HT. However, the other benefits of transdermal delivery outweigh this small drawback.

The 2008 Danish Sex Hormone Register Study confirmed what I have been saying for years about transdermal estrogen and cyclic oral progesterone. This is the first large-scale observational study that addresses the influence of various regimens, doses, and delivery systems. The researchers found that transdermal estrogen did lower the risk of heart disease while they found that continuous combined oral estrogen-progesterone regimens such as the one used in the WHI trial were associated with higher risks.

BIO-IDENTICAL PREPARATIONS
MADE BY COMPOUNDING PHARMACIES

Along with the mass retreat from HT that happened in the wake of the 2002 Premarin and Prempro scare when the WHI study was stopped, a lot of women jumped on the bio-identical hormone bandwagon. However, instead of taking the FDA-approved brands made by drug companies as I did, many women got prescriptions from their physicians based on the results of saliva tests. These prescriptions purportedly customize the hormone dosages to suit any given woman's needs. The problem with that approach is two-fold. First, the saliva tests are unreliable. Second, the preparations mixed by the compounding pharmacists have never been tested for safety or efficacy. Ironically, proponents of the bio-identicals made by compounding pharmacies often claim that these preparations are safer because they are "natural." That's such a comforting word but there's no proof to back up the claim. Again, let me underscore that what does make a difference is the delivery system and dose. Transdermal wins hands down over oral as far as I'm concerned.

SHOULD MENOPAUSE BE "MEDICALIZED"?

Yet another response to the WHI scare was the emergence of a school of thought that says menopause is a natural event in a woman's life that shouldn't be "medicalized" and that women should simply avoid hormones at all costs. I don't buy that. My stance is that if you are in the throes of menopause, don't hesitate to talk to your doctor about the pros and cons of HT given your unique medical history. The final word on the benefits of HT at menopause for some women has not yet been spoken.

There's no one-size-fits-all answer. Whenever I hear people insist that menopause is a natural event that shouldn't be "medicalized," I can't help but think about one of my patients. Diana was forty-three when she came to me and said, "Please, please, turn off the water! I totally soak the sheets with night sweats and I get barely any sleep. My husband ends up on the couch half the time. We hardly ever have sex anymore and my moods are all over the place. I have trouble concentrating at the office and I have a hot flash like every other minute during the day. I can't go on like this for another ten years! Help!"

I did help her. She was not at high risk for breast cancer so I felt she was someone for whom HT, especially transdermal, was an option for which the benefits would outweigh any slight risks. In a situation like Diana's, I see absolutely no need to tell her to tough it out. Margaret Mead's proclamation about "menopausal zest" notwithstanding, Diana

Will the Patch "Sweat Off"?

No. I promise you from personal experience that it stays on even when you're dripping after a workout or soaking in a hot tub. The patch is barely visible and blends into your skin. Wear it on your lower abdomen area within the panty line. I rotate sites and wash off the adhesive residue using a little moisturizer.

Do I Ever Need to Interrupt
My Hormone Therapy?

Yes. For a small number of women on HT, their breast density may increase slightly and for that reason stopping hormones a few weeks before a mammogram can be necessary in order to get an accurate test result. Even more important, you need to stop your HT for several weeks prior to surgery to prevent the possibility of blood clots.

was miserable to the point that her marriage and her job performance were suffering. For someone like her, HT is the only remedy that really works to relieve the most severe symptoms.

Having said that, if you're in the 80 percent who could use some relief, I strongly recommend that you ask your doctor about the transdermal method I prefer and prescribe. I have had patients resist me by saying that the patch seems like too much trouble or doesn't appeal to them because it's visible to the men in their lives and might be something of a turn-off. These seem like very weak arguments given the health benefits of transdermal delivery over oral delivery. However, if you absolutely don't want to try the patch, then ask about some of the newer and lower-dose oral estrogen and progesterone products. The most frequently prescribed combination still consists of conjugated equine estrogen tablets (brand name Premarin) and medroxyprogesterone acetate (MPA) tablets (brand name Provera). The dose of CEE in most HT regimens is now typically 0.625 mg or 0.3 mg. The MPA is usually given in a dosage of 10 mg for ten to twelve days a month. Some physicians give the MPA in a lower dose such as 5 mg or only once every second or third month to decrease the incidence of PMS-like effects. However, there's a trade-off in that the protection of the uterine lining is lessened, although if your estrogen dose is only 0.3 mg, this is rarely a concern.

Additional formulations of estrogen and progesterone have been developed and are often substituted these days for Premarin and Provera. Micronized estradiol (brand name Estrace) is a bio-identical drug that was approved by the FDA in 1993. It is made from a plant source and has the hypothetical advantage of actually being estradiol, the bio-active form of estrogen, although the micronized oral drug is altered by the liver just as any other oral preparation would be. In this case, the estradiol turns into a weaker form of estrogen called estrone. Some other brands of oral estrogen preparations include Ogen and Estratab. There is also a new oral HT called Angelique, but long-term safety has not yet been established. The transdermal CombiPatch delivers the

Are Birth Control Pills a Good Option for Menopausal Women?

No, although some doctors assure perimenopausal women the pills are safe and can be taken right up to menopause. The trouble is that the amount of estrogen and progesterone required to shut down ovulation is too high for a woman whose ovulation is already shutting down on its own. Taking the Pill to regulate the erratic, heavy periods typical of perimenopause does work, and, of course, it also protects you against unplanned pregnancies. However, as I found out when I took the Pill to manage heavy periods in my mid-forties, there are risks even with a low-dose version of the Pill. My blood pressure went up for the first time in my life. It went back down again after I stopped the Pill. I eventually switched to HT when I began experiencing insomnia and nighttime hot flashes and that controlled my symptoms without raising my blood pressure. Also, no woman who smokes should consider the Pill. The risks of blood clots, heart attacks, and strokes are too high.

same estradiol as other patches but also contains a synthetic progestin, which I don't recommend. Both Angelique and the CombiPatch not only have synthetic progestins but they also deliver the progestins continuously. I prefer the transdermal estrogen along with cyclical use of the oral micronized progesterone, Prometrium. It seems to cause fewer PMS-like symptoms in women who are sensitive to progestin, and it's bio-identical so it produces none of the androgenic side effects. It is distributed in 100 or 200 mg capsules and is usually given in a dose of 200 mg for ten to twelve days a month. So far micronized progesterone is only available as an oral medication. Pharmaceutical companies are having difficulty manufacturing a delivery system for transdermal progesterone that is consistent and predictable. There are also ongoing studies using intravaginal progesterone in postmenopausal women but the results have not yet been published.

In the end, only you can decide what's right for you. Listen to your body. If the method of HT you're using works, stick with it. If you're getting annoying symptoms such as heavy bleeding, you may not be taking enough progesterone or you may be inadvertently skipping doses. Another possibility is that you're making quite a bit of endogenous (internal) estrogen in your visceral fat. This may sound good but it's not. For one thing, you're no longer making endogenous progesterone to balance out the endogenous estrogen, and for another, the bleeding is a tip-off to your doctor that you're carrying a dangerous amount of belly fat that can lead to metabolic syndrome or worse. You don't need to be taking more exogenous (from an external source) estrogen on top of what you're making. You need to lose weight and get your waist measurement under thirty-five inches or at least lose one or two inches. That will be enough to make a big difference to your future health risk! Sorry to sound like a scold, but this is so vital. I'll help you out when we get to chapter 11.

The bottom line is that each woman should stay attuned to how she feels and what is or isn't working for her and tailor her choices accordingly.

HEALTH STRATEGIES TO
HELP YOU LIVE LONG AND WELL

Whether you breeze through menopause with minimal complaints or you suffer from every symptom in the book, your body will be different when the process is complete, as we have seen. This is true, by the way, even if taking HT gives you the illusion that you're still menstruating. HT doesn't do anything to slow down or reverse the aging of your reproductive system, or any other system for that matter. Years ago HT was touted as an elixir of youth, but while it may do a little something to stave off wrinkles, it can't keep you forever young. In fact, lifestyle measures—my mantra, the "Lifestyle Pill"!—such as diet, exercise (especially weight-bearing), getting enough sleep, minimizing alcohol consumption, and wearing sunscreen and wide-brimmed hats will do more in the end to give you the good looks and vigor that will belie your age. My "Lifestyle Pill" is still better than any other pill or medication we have to offer for keeping you humming along with good health, good spirits, and good looks!

Here's what I recommend:

- Know your baseline bone density (see chapter 3, page 116).
- Take 1,200 mg of calcium daily.
- Take at least 1,000 IU of vitamin D daily. (This is based on new research about the many benefits of increased amounts of vitamin D, especially for postmenopausal women.)
- Keep your waist measurement under thirty-five inches. (See chapter 11 for tips on how to do this with exercise and good nutrition.)
- Know your C-reactive protein, triglyceride level, cholesterol level, and breakdown (see chapter 3, pages 107–8).
- Know your blood pressure and keep it below 130/80 with lifestyle measures and possibly medication.

- If you're at high risk for heart disease because of family history or because you smoke, have high C-reactive protein, or have abnormal blood fats such as high LDL cholesterol and/or low HDL cholesterol and high triglycerides, talk with your doctor about a special cardiac test that measures your calcium score on a CT scan.
- Have a colonoscopy at age fifty.
- Take cat naps. Researchers from Harvard School of Public Health found that midday naps reduced coronary death by about one-third in women.
- Try acupuncture. Research results are inconclusive, but some studies suggest that acupuncture works well in relieving menopausal symptoms.
- Try daily fish oil capsules, particularly if you are at risk for heart disease. They are chock-full of healthful omega-3s—I take two to four capsules daily. I don't have "hard" proof yet of the benefits, but evidence is mounting that more omega-3s are important for so many vital functions.

BEHIND CLOSED DOORS: THE BEST SEX NOW

As we age, the need for intimacy, connectedness, and some type of sexual activity actually increases. So do the benefits of sex. Also, as many of us have discovered to our delight, menopause often ushers in an era when lovemaking can be more spontaneous and spicy than ever before. Long-married couples eventually have the house and their free time all to themselves after decades of fitting in sex around the kids' needs and schedules. Suddenly single women often report that being free at last from concerns about unplanned pregnancies adds extra sizzle to the dating scene. Some of them find themselves involved with men several years their junior—the so-called cougar-and-cub phenomenon. As one of my patients confided, "He's forty-five and pre-Viagra. I'm fifty-four and post menopausal with no need for birth control. We got ourselves checked for STIs so we aren't even using condoms. We just can't keep our hands off each other. I've never had so much fun in my life!"

However, she wouldn't have been having all that fun without a little help from modern medicine. She was my patient for a reason. She had come to me early in the relationship with the new man in her life because she was, as she put it, "not juicy down there anymore." Her first attempts at sex with him were painful. Also, penetration was difficult. I wasn't surprised. One of the most common features of the postmenopausal body is a condition called atrophic vaginitis. When estrogen levels decrease, the tissues of the vagina and the labia become thinner and drier. Even when a woman is sexually aroused, she may have soreness and she may not have enough lubrication.

I know whereof I speak. The symptoms of atrophic vaginitis sneak up on you. In retrospect I can't come up with a precise time of the onset of this condition for me, but over a few years time, I had noticed a change in my vulvar and vaginal tissues and my comfort with sex. Since this was so subtle at first, it was not until I was finally treated and suddenly felt normal again that I realized how compromised sex had been. My sex "life" was still great and frequent, but "sex" per se was compromised because of the worry about pain. I still seemed to have some lubrication with sex although that too had diminished somewhat.

As recently as 2001 a Gallup poll showed that by the average age of fifty-seven, 50 percent of women had stopped having sex for a number of different reasons, one of the most common being pain with intercourse because of a dry vagina. Yet when the women who reported vaginal dryness were asked whether there was anything that could be done about the problem, 90 percent of them responded that there was not. Oh, but there is! I'll tell you all about it. But first I'll tell you how to be sure that you do have atrophic vaginitis.

TESTS FOR ATROPHIC VAGINITIS

- Your Pap smear result is often the earliest clue. The cells under the microscope may show an increased proportion of parabasal cells and a decreased percentage of superficial cells. Take a look at the copy of your Pap smear report. Does it say something about abnormal cells consistent with atrophic vaginitis or inadequate or low estrogen effect? It could also show, as mine did, what is called an "ASCUS" result. (Note: ASCUS in young women is more often due to an HPV infection, whereas in older women it is commonly caused by low estrogen.)
- If you test your vaginal pH with a home test kit, it may be high, usually over five, because of the loss of estrogen. (See chapter 7, page 203.)

CYTOPATHOLOGY REPORT   CG05-802!

INTERPRETATION/RESULT:

GYNECOLOGICAL SPECIMEN, CERVICAL/ENDOCERVICAL, THIN PREP:

ATYPICAL SQUAMOUS CELLS OF UNDETERMINED SIGNIFICANCE (ASC-US), SQUAMOUS ATYPIA.
  -Marked inflammation present.

Adequacy: SATISFACTORY FOR EVALUATION
  -Endocervical/Transformation zone component present.

NOTE: Cervical/Vaginal cytology is a screening test primarily for squamous cancers and precursors and has been associated with false negative and false positive results. New technologies, such as liquid-based sampling, may decrease, but will not eliminate, all false results. Regular sampling and follow-up of clinically unexplained signs and symptoms are recommended to minimize false negative results.

Moira D. Wood, M.D.
Report Electronically Signed

This diagnostic report has been personally interpreted by the signatory of report.

P.JF/PJF/CH/SMA/MDW/MDW /PJF .
CH

Source of Specimen:
GYNECOLOGICAL SPECIMEN, CERVICAL/ENDOCERVICAL, THIN PREP

PAP STAIN/THIN PREP Received: 1

Clinical Diagnosis and History
Date of Last Menstrual Period: UNKNOWN
Other Clinical Conditions: Squamous Atypia, within one year: 3/04
HPV DNA HIGH RISK TEST – NOT DETECTED.

Pap test results suggesting atrophic vaginitis

- An intravaginal ultrasound to measure the uterine lining will show a very thin atrophic endometrium between four and five mm.

TREATING ATROPHIC VAGINITIS

Sexual activity itself is just what the doctor ordered. In addition to all the other health benefits covered in chapter 2, sex has been shown to increase vaginal elasticity and lubrication. However, sex does nothing to restore or maintain estrogen levels, so you will almost certainly need some help, as my "cougar" patient and I did, in getting past the pain.

Estrogen Replacement

Taking some form of estrogen is an incredibly effective treatment. Estrogen restores normal pH levels and thickens the vaginal, urethral, and vulvar tissues. Estrogen will also increase the number of superficial cells seen on the Pap smear, and therefore your Pap smear may now report "normal estrogen effect." In addition to the HRT options detailed in this chapter, you may also want to consider intravaginal tablets, creams, gels, or rings. Your vaginal tissues—and your sex partner—will thank you. I know. I've been there! Also, I've been prescribing estrogen cream for my patients with atrophic vaginitis for years.

You could notice a difference in a few weeks' time, although you may need a few months to feel normal again. Women who have severe atrophic vaginitis have a diminished blood supply to the vaginal tissues so that at first not much estrogen gets absorbed systemically. As the tissues improve, the blood supply does as well. Eventually more estrogen gets absorbed. The level is so low that you probably won't need to take progesterone to balance out the lining of your endometrium. Even a woman with prior breast cancer can use small intravaginal doses of estrogen for comfortable sex as long as her oncologist agrees. On occasion, doctors will prescribe a ten-day course of progesterone and wait for the response. If no vaginal bleeding occurs, then it is likely that the little bit of topical estrogen is not affecting the uterus. If bleeding does

Topical Estrogen by Cream, Tablet, Gel, and Rings

- Estrace, cream, 1.0 mg estradiol
- Premarin, cream, 0.625 mg conjugated estrogens/g
- Ogen, cream, 1.5 mg estropipate
- Vagifem, vaginal tablets, 25 mcg estradiol
- Estring, vaginal ring, 0.075 mg/day estradiol
- Femring, vaginal ring, 0.05, 0.10 mg/day estradiol acetate
- EstroGel, gel, 1.25 gm/day delivering 0.75 mg estradiol
- Estrasorb, emulsion (cream), 0.05 mg estradiol

Estrogen cream is usually inserted via an applicator daily for two weeks and then twice weekly or as needed to treat the symptoms. The sustained-release estradiol ring is replaced every ninety days. The estradiol tablet is usually inserted deep inside the vagina once daily for two weeks, and the dose is then decreased to twice weekly.

occur, which suggests higher-than-expected systemic levels of estrogen from fat cells, your doctor will probably recommend that you take intermittent progesterone along with the intravaginal estrogen after other possible causes, such as cancer, have been ruled out.

Other Treatments

Lubricants

Lubricants do nothing to thicken, strengthen, or repair vaginal tissue. They provide lubrication or slipperiness only for a brief time after they are inserted, so they do make sex more comfortable. Many women try lubricants before making a decision about topical hormone treatment or they use lubricants while waiting for the hormones to kick in or to supplement the topical hormones.

- Water-based vaginal lubricants, such as K-Y Jelly, are inexpensive and work great. There are many generic brands at your local pharmacy. Just make sure the label says "water soluble." Petroleum-based products such as petrolatum or petroleum jelly can break down latex condoms, increase the risk of vaginal infections, and form a barrier so that water-soluble lubricants or your own natural lubricants won't work. They quickly lose their lubricating ability as soon as they are warmed up in the body or on the hands. I tell my patients to keep the lubricant in the refrigerator although even that doesn't help for very long after you apply the product.
- Replens Vaginal Moisturizer, a popular water-soluble lubricant, is advertised to work for two to three days after a single application.
- Vitamin E capsules or suppositories inserted into the vagina about three times per week apparently work quite well.

A final word about sex and the menopausal woman: If you think your sex life is just fine, it is. A 2008 study done by Massachusetts General Hospital showed that while close to 45 percent of the women in the study reported issues such as low desire or orgasm difficulties, only 12 percent of them overall and only 8.9 percent of those over sixty-five said the problems caused them distress. The researchers concluded that labeling the women who reported no distress as being sexually dysfunctional would be inappropriate. Was it good for you? That's good enough!

Now we've completed Part II and you know all about the three seasons of your life as a woman. Many of the world's religions, ancient and modern, have versions of the Triple Goddess. One of these is the Apaches' Changing Woman that you learned about in chapter 4. Nice concept! We all ought to celebrate the miracle of our tripartite feminine existence. Even so, glorifying those womanly deities doesn't address one little detail: Goddesses are immune to the problems "down there" that can plague us flesh-and-blood females. In Part III, I'll teach you about vaginal, bowel, and urinary troubles. You'll find frank explanations and real solutions. What are you waiting for? Turn the page!

PART III

Is This Normal or Should I Call My Doctor?

7

"Female Problems" from Cause to Cure

IN THIS CHAPTER

- Vaginitis

- Fibroids

- Endometriosis

- Pelvic Inflammatory Disease (PID)

- Vulvodynia

- Gynecologic Cancers

- Hysterectomies

Back in chapter 1, you learned about the inner workings and healthy functioning of your female reproductive organs. This chapter lists for you the many things that can go wrong with those organs. Several of the problems are serious, but most of them fall into the nuisance category. They're so common that it's fair to say that all of us will experience at least one of them at some point in our lives. I'll share with you what I've learned from my twenty-five years of caring for women and from my own experiences with "female problems." I've had just about every vaginal infection there is! I got my first yeast infection way back when I was in medical school. Bacterial vaginosis hit right after I got married and then I had to deal with another bout of BV as a postmenopausal woman. Along the way I had occasional yeast infections after taking antibiotics, and today I'm on hormone therapy to treat atrophic vaginitis. When it comes to embarrassing itches and discharges "down there,"

I can honestly say I know firsthand what works, what doesn't, when you need a doctor, and when you can treat yourself.

Fortunately, though, I've been spared the more worrisome gynecological disorders. However, I've treated countless patients with those problems. I can give you advice about what course to take if you do contract a condition that is life-threatening or that puts your fertility in jeopardy or that simply causes unrelenting pain. I'll be speaking to you from the heart both as a woman and as a doctor while I point you toward the best possible outcomes. I want to keep you from making hasty decisions about your treatment options out of fear or lack of knowledge. As always, my philosophy is that *you* are the most important member of your health-care team. You have every right to ask questions, get a second or third opinion, do your own research, and allow your "health radar" to be your guide.

That said, let's leave the scary issues until later in the chapter and begin instead with the garden variety problems that you're most likely to encounter.

VAGINITIS

Vaginitis happens when the natural, healthy balance of bacteria in the vagina is upset because unfriendly bacteria of various types manage to overpower the good guys. The term is a catch-all diagnosis for any inflammation of the vagina or vulvar area. The medical suffix "itis" means "inflammation." An inflammation can be caused by an infection or by allergies and abrasions. An inflamed area is typically warm, swollen, and red. Vaginitis usually also involves pain or itching and an abnormal discharge.

About 90 percent of vaginitis cases are caused by one of three infections: bacterial vaginosis (BV), a yeast infection, or trichomoniasis. The other 10 percent are noninfectious. I'll discuss BV, yeast, and noninfectious vaginitis in this chapter. Turn to the section on sexually transmitted infections (STIs) in chapter 2 to read about trichomoniasis.

201

BACTERIAL VAGINOSIS (BV)

Bacterial vaginosis is the cause of over 50 percent of all cases of vaginitis. BV was originally called "nonspecific vaginitis," but in 1984 a team of researchers coined the current term using the medical suffix that means "disease." About half of all women who get BV have no significant symptoms, and the condition may simply go away on its own. However, any woman with symptoms should see a doctor. Left untreated, BV can cause pelvic inflammatory disease (see the section on PID later in this chapter) or chronic pelvic pain. Untreated infections also lower a woman's

---

What's the Best Way to Keep My Genital Area Clean?

Right after my first son was born, I discovered that the hypoallergenic baby wipes I had bought for him were also perfect for keeping my own "private parts" clean. The French have the bidet and at least one American company is now making a toilet seat that doubles as a bidet, but I simply use my wipes. They're soothing, effective, and portable. I keep containers of them in the bathrooms and the powder room in my house and I carry a travel-size packet in my purse.

Toilet paper is dry and irritating. It doesn't cleanse your vulvar area well at all. In fact, a report published in the prestigious *Journal of the American Medical Association* confirms this. Think about all that happens in such a small area "down there"—we have sex, we urinate, and we have bowel movements. Baby wipes clean best and they moisturize delicate tissues. My personal favorites are wipes infused with aloe, but use any brand that feels good to you. However, stay away from scented wipes that can cause allergic reactions. Also, even if your brand claims to be "flushable," don't risk backing up the plumbing.

natural defenses against other infections including HIV (see chapter 2, page 65), and increase the risk of miscarriage and preterm labor in pregnant women. In addition, BV seems to increase the risk of infections after hysterectomies and abortions. In fact BV is enough of a concern that some specialists recommend that all women who are pregnant or scheduled for gynecologic surgery be treated for BV as a prophylactic measure.

How to Tell if You Have Bacterial Vaginosis

Early Symptoms

- thin whitish-gray discharge
- fishy odor
- itching in the vulvar and vaginal area
- burning during urination

Advanced Symptoms

Stomachaches or cramps that are not related to your period may signal that a formerly "silent" (symptomless) BV infection has spread. Call your doctor if you have stomachaches or cramps.

Diagnostic Tests You Can Buy over the Counter

Over-the-counter pH tests are now available in most grocery stores and pharmacies. A high pH indicates an upset of the acid/alkaline balance in the vagina. The abbreviation "pH" stands for "power of hydrogen." The concept was introduced in 1909 by the Danish chemist S. P. L. Sørensen as a measure of the activity of hydrogen ions in a solution.

If you find that your pH is abnormally high, that's a tip-off that you may have BV or trichomoniasis (see chapter 2, page 73). Make an appointment with your gynecologist for further testing. (As noted earlier, blood—including menstrual blood—and semen can raise the

Do Not Douche!

I suspect that nothing tempts a woman to douche more than the embarrassing fishy odor that is the most prevalent symptom of BV, especially right after sex. Yet ironically, douching can *cause* BV and also make it worse by further upsetting the balance of healthy and harmful bacteria. Douching is a very bad idea! Don't do it.

pH temporarily. Don't use the self-tests during your period or after sex.)

Diagnostic Tests That Require an Office Visit

Your doctor will do a gynecological exam using a speculum and a swab (see chapter 3) to get tissue samples that will be sent to a laboratory. The samples will be tested for the following:

- the so-called "clue cells" characteristic of BV
- the release of a fishy odor (the "whiff test")
- a high pH

Causes of Bacterial Vaginosis

Men don't get BV because they don't have vaginas, so you can't "catch" BV from a man. However, having sex with a male partner can bring on a BV episode for a woman. This is because our vaginas are naturally acidic while semen is alkaline. Men who have had vasectomies still have semen that is alkaline because all that's missing is the sperm. The main bacteria in the vagina, lactobacilli, can be overwhelmed when the acidic environment in which they thrive becomes more alkaline due to the presence of semen. This allows unfriendly bacteria to grow. Because your body responds differently to the semen of different men, the risk of

Treating Bacterial Vaginosis

The two reasons to treat BV are to relieve your symptoms and to reduce the chances of future problems.

Medications for Bacterial Vaginosis

I always prefer the most targeted and least systemic treatment so as not to cause secondary problems by wiping out or disturbing the natural balance of bacteria in other parts of the body. Here are my recommendations:

- Flagyl/Metrogel vaginal suppository
- metronidazole gel, 0.75 percent, one full applicator (5g) intravaginally, once a day for 5 days
- clindamycin cream, 2 percent, one full applicator (5g) intravaginally at bedtime for 7 days. (Warning: Clindamycin cream is oil-based. That means it could weaken diaphragms and latex condoms for up to five days after you stop using the medication.)

In addition, here are the commonly prescribed antibiotics for BV. If your doctor suggests one of these, why not ask whether a topical remedy can be substituted?

- metronidazole 500 mg orally twice a day for 7 days
- Flagyl/Metrogel in pill or gel form, 500 mg twice a day for 7 days. (Avoid drinking *any* alcohol during treatment and for twenty-four hours after your last dose. Combining even small amounts of alcohol with Flagyl can make you very sick to your stomach, and may even cause vomiting.)
- clindamycin 300 mg orally twice a day for 7 days
- clindamycin ovules 100 mg intravaginally once at bedtime for 3 days

YEAST INFECTIONS

Now we come to the problem most women associate with vaginitis: yeast infections. Anyone who's had an episode of this incredibly itchy and

Why Did the Results of My Pap Smear Mention Yeast?

Pap smears often show false-positive results for yeast. If you read your Pap smear results as I encourage you to do and you see a reference to yeast, this does *not* mean you have an infection but rather that the yeast is living happily among your other vaginal bacteria. There's no need to do anything unless you develop symptoms.

sometimes painful annoyance dreads a recurrence. Seventy-five percent of all women have at least one episode of yeast vaginitis in their lifetime. However, according to a study done by Susan Hoffstetter, Ph.D., of the Saint Louis University School of Medicine, only 26 percent of women who believed they had yeast infections were correct. That's why you need either a home test or a visit to the doctor to be sure of the diagnosis even if you have what you think are pretty clear symptoms.

How to Tell If You Have a Yeast Infection
Symptoms

- intense itching in the vulvar area
- a white, odorless discharge that has curds
- burning and pain during urination
- pain during sex

Diagnostic Tests You Can Buy over the Counter
Self-test kits from the grocery store or drugstore can help you determine whether your infection may be yeast or something else. Yeast infections typically don't result in a high pH, whereas BV (discussed earlier in this chapter) and "trich" (see chapter 2) do. If your pH is low, meaning normal,

One Woman's Story: Jennifer, Age 28

"I swear I get my period every time my boyfriend and I go on a camping trip no matter when I'm actually supposed to get it. The last time we went camping, I decided to use panty liners just in case. I had recently lost ten pounds so I was really psyched about fitting into a new pair of skinny jeans and I didn't want to stain them. So anyway, the morning of the third day, there we were in the woods in a tent in the pouring rain when I woke up with the most insane itching in my vagina. I just wanted to dig at it but scratching didn't help at all. There was also a disgusting discharge. It didn't smell but it was definitely yucky. This had never happened to me before and I freaked out.

"There was no cell signal so I couldn't call my doctor. I finally told my boyfriend what was going on and he said we should hike out until we got a signal. My doctor's staff relayed his message that he was almost positive I had a yeast infection. He said my vagina probably stayed too wet because of the panty liners and the tight jeans, not to mention the soggy weather conditions. We kept going until we got to a little town that had a drugstore that carried the cream my doctor recommended. I didn't even need a prescription and the itching and discharge went away in about a week. Next time I'll skip the panty liners and wear my comfy old cargo pants!"

you can safely try one of the many effective yeast medications that can be purchased without a prescription. I've done this several times myself with success. If your pH is high, meaning abnormal, make an appointment with your doctor to get a correct diagnosis and the best treatment.

Diagnostic Tests That Require an Office Visit

Your doctor will do a physical exam to look for signs of a yeast infection. Symptoms, also called subjective findings, are what you experience firsthand. Signs, also called objective evidence, are what your doctor observes or measures.

Your doctor may see any or all of the following:

- swelling of the vulva
- fissures or cracks in the skin
- excoriations or raw areas of the vulva skin
- the characteristic "curdy" vaginal discharge

Your doctor can also do the following tests

- She can examine the vaginal discharge by adding a drop of salt water (saline) to vaginal discharge on a slide and using a microscope to search for causes of infection other than yeast.
- She can add a little 10 percent potassium hydroxide (KOH) to another slide with your vaginal discharge and take a look under the microscope. The solution improves the visualization of yeast by dissolving surrounding cellular material that might obscure the yeast. However, as many as 30 percent of symptomatic yeast infections have false-negative KOH results.
- She can do what is called a Gram stain of the vaginal discharge, which means applying a special stain to the smear on a slide to look for budding yeast called pseudohyphae.
- If you have a recurrent problem, she may also do a culture for yeast species to find out exactly what type of yeast is present, if any.

Causes of Yeast Infections

The culprit is a fungus called Candida albicans. It normally lives in the vagina, mouth, and digestive tract without causing any problems. Under certain circumstances Candida can "overgrow" and change from a harmless, one-cell fungus into long branches, or hyphae, with budding spores called mycelia. The full medical term for this condition is

What Can I Do to Clear Up My Yeast Infection Faster?

These are simple steps you can take to speed your recovery and keep infections from recurring:

1. Don't use tampons while you're being treated for a yeast infection.

2. Even after the infection is gone, don't use super absorbent tampons.

3. While you're being treated, change your sanitary pads frequently.

4. Wear cotton underwear, or panties and pantyhose with cotton crotches. Synthetic fabrics don't wick up moisture. That leads to "maceration" or "soaking and softening" of tissues. This in turn encourages fungal overgrowth.

5. Don't wear tight jeans.

6. Use baby wipes after each bowel movement. Be sure to wipe from front to back.

7. Do not douche.

8. If you use a diaphragm, rinse it off after each use and never leave it in for days at a time as I once did when I was on call as a medical resident.

9. Don't stop taking or applying your prescribed medication just because you feel better. If you do, you may increase the chance of the infection coming back.

vulvovaginal candidiasis or VCC. Symptoms often begin just before the start of your period. If you have a history of recurring infections, ask your doctor whether you could benefit from a prescription for a medication to be taken preventively once a month.

Yeast, or Candida, is not "caught" from a sexual partner. Women who have never had sex are just as susceptible. I am thinking of the nuns who are my patients. I have treated many of the sisters for yeast infections over the years.

Conditions that could make you more susceptible to yeast infections:

- antibiotics, especially with frequent use
- metabolic syndrome
- diabetes
- pregnancy
- chemotherapy (see sidebar on page 213)
- HIV
- birth control pills
- tight jeans and panty hose that prevent your genital area from airing out
- panty liners worn 24/7, thus keeping the genital area too moist
- synthetic fabrics that don't absorb moisture

Treatments for Yeast Infections

Back when I had my first yeast infection in the 1970s, I was stuck with one treatment: inserting into my vagina a yellow tablet that leaked out all over my underwear. Now we have many readily available, safe, and effective ways to treat yeast infections, both by prescription and over the counter.

Unfortunately, some women suspect yeast every time they have vaginal symptoms such as itching and discharge. They're tempted to start OTC treatment for yeast although they may have a different infection instead. That's why I'm a fan of the simple vaginal pH self-tests, described earlier

Why Do I Have Vaginal Infections Now That I'm on Chemotherapy?

Doctors often fail to warn women who are undergoing treatment for cancer that they will be at increased risk for vaginal complaints. Here's what you need to know:

- Chemotherapy and estrogen-blocking hormones such as tamoxifen or Arimidex can cause atrophic vaginitis.
- These treatments also compromise your immune system so that you have fewer white blood cells to fight vaginal infections.
- You may be given antibiotics and this can heighten your risk of vaginal infections.

in this chapter. If your pH is high, make an appointment with your doctor. However, no harm is done if you treat yourself for yeast while you're waiting for your doctor's appointment. It's possible to have a yeast infection along with another problem that is causing the high pH. Treatment for yeast won't mask any other conditions and if you do have a yeast infection as well as something else, you'll have gotten a head start on curing it.

Medications for Yeast Infections
Topical Applications
The creams and suppositories are usually oil-based and might weaken latex condoms and diaphragms. Topical agents usually cause no serious side effects although local burning or irritation might occur.

- butoconazole 2 percent cream, 5 g intravaginally for 3 days
- butoconazole 2 percent cream, 5 g single intravaginal application

- clotrimazole 1 percent cream, 5 g intravaginally for 7 to 14 days
- clotrimazole 100 mg vaginal tablet for 7 days
- clotrimazole 100 mg vaginal tablet, two tablets for 3 days
- miconazole 2 percent cream, 5 g intravaginally for 7 days
- miconazole 100 mg vaginal suppository, one suppository for 7 days
- miconazole 200 mg vaginal suppository, one suppository for 3 days
- miconazole 1,200 mg vaginal suppository, one suppository for 1 day
- nystatin 100,000-unit vaginal tablet, one tablet for 14 days
- Tioconazole 6.5 percent ointment, 5 g intravaginally in a single application
- Terconazole 0.4 percent cream, 5 g intravaginally for 7 days
- Terconazole 0.8 percent cream, 5 g intravaginally for 3 days
- Terconazole 80 mg vaginal suppository, one suppository for 3 days

Pills

Oral medication always poses a greater risk of adverse effects. Also, pills are usually more expensive than topical treatments. Still, more and more women are asking for oral treatments because they don't want

Can I Have Sex While I'm Being Treated for A Yeast Infection?

You run the risk of infecting your partner's scrotal skin during intercourse. He can wear a condom but that won't protect the entire area. If he does end up with symptoms, including itching and redness, topical antifungal medications can clear up the condition. Ultimately, the decision of whether or not to have sex is up to the two of you. If you don't experience any pain and your partner is willing, go ahead. I hesitate to tell people to abstain when no real harm will be done.

Is It True That Boric Acid Can Cure a Yeast Infection?

Boric acid is an incredibly effective treatment for yeast infections. We're not sure why, but it may alter the vaginal pH so that the environment is less friendly to yeast. Doses of 600/650 mg capsule inserted deep into the vagina once or twice daily for two weeks or so works well. Boric acid can also be used during the second half of the menstrual cycle to prevent yeast infections in women with frequent recurrences. Boric acid does require a prescription, however, and it can be irritating to delicates tissues. *Warning:* Boric acid is toxic if taken orally.

to be bothered inserting potentially messy creams or tablets. The only approved pill is fluconazole (Diflucan), 150 mg oral tablet, one tablet in a single dose.

NONINFECTIOUS VAGINITIS

Inflammations of the vulva (vulvitis) and the vagina are not always caused by infections. Here are the other perpetrators:

Allergies

Allergic vaginitis can be caused by soaps, detergents, powders, dyes, synthetic fabrics, perfumed sanitary pads, bubble baths, and perfumed douches.

Abrasions

Rough washcloths and toilet paper can create tiny cracks or fissures in delicate skin. Single-ply toilet paper is actually better than two-ply, however, because the softer version can "ball up" so that small pieces are left behind. (See my advice about baby wipes earlier in this chapter.)

Overly Moist Genital Area

Some of the offenders are tight jeans, pantyhose, synthetic fabrics, and worn panty liners twenty-four/seven.

Atrophic Vaginitis

This is a condition that affects menopausal women as their estrogen levels decline. The vulva and vagina shrink or atrophy. Atrophic vaginitis is painful but it does not usually cause vaginal discharge. It's not a bacterial infection or even an inflammation as the "itis" suffix would suggest. I have diagnosed and treated hundreds of women with atrophic vaginitis over the past twenty-five years, and I recently learned firsthand what a painful and troubling condition it is! Turn to chapter 6 for a complete discussion of this problem.

Now you know how to take charge of your health if you contract any version of the nuisance ailment collectively called vaginitis. Next I'm going to give you a crash course in the "female problems" that can be serious. Home remedies and lifestyle changes won't prevent or treat these conditions, but that doesn't mean you're powerless. On the contrary, you remain the one who is most keenly attuned to symptoms, if any, and you are still a full partner in your health care regarding decisions about your treatment options.

If you suspect you have any of the disorders that I'll detail on the following pages of this chapter, let your doctor know. Should you get a positive diagnosis, you can take it upon yourself to research both traditional and alternative therapies and discuss them with your doctor. Remaining proactive about your health concerns is never more important than when the stakes are high. This is no time to fall back into "Yes, Doctor" mode. And if you're too sick or too scared to speak up for yourself, call on your health buddy for support and help. Remember, I'm rooting for you. I know from experience that patients who never forget that they are the most important members of their health-care team are those who have the best chance of optimal outcomes.

FIBROIDS

Uterine fibroids, also called leiomyomas, are noncancerous tumors. Fibroids typically appear during the childbearing years and shrink after menopause. About one-quarter of Caucasian women and as many as half of African-American women have fibroids. In the majority of cases, the growths are so small that they cause no symptoms and no problems. For example, I had no idea I had a fibroid until it showed up on a routine ultrasound. My fibroid was so inconsequential that the doctor didn't even mention it to me, but I read my own report and saw the note referring to the incidental fibroid. However, some women have large fibroids that cause heavy menstrual bleeding and painful cramps. These women often end up with severe anemia. Fibroids can also reduce a woman's chances of getting pregnant if they are in a position that blocks the fallopian tubes. In women who do get pregnant, large fibroids can compete with the fetus for blood supply.

HOW TO TELL IF YOU HAVE FIBROIDS
Symptoms

- dysmenorrhea, meaning unusually painful menstrual periods
- menorrhagia, meaning very heavy bleeding during menstrual periods
- sudden, acute pelvic pain if a fibroid outgrows its blood supply (This is rare but when it happens the pain can be severe. Call your doctor immediately.)
- low back pain
- leg pain
- stress incontinence (see chapter 9, page 290)
- constipation (see chapter 8, page 237)

Diagnostic Tests

- blood test to check for iron-deficiency anemia caused by excessive blood loss
- ultrasound
- hysterosonography, a type of ultrasound in which a saline solution is used to expand the uterus
- hysterosalpingography, an X-ray that uses a dye to show images of the uterus and fallopian tubes. (See chapter 9 for information about allergic reactions to X-ray dyes.)
- hysteroscopy with a thin lighted scope placed inside your uterus

TYPES OF FIBROIDS

Some are inside the uterine wall, others are outside it, and still others grow on stalks inside the uterus. The latter can twist and cut off their own blood supply causing acute pain.

CAUSES OF FIBROIDS

No one knows for sure what causes fibroids. However, because fibroids contain more estrogen than the rest of the uterine wall, researchers speculate that the extra estrogen and progesterone produced during pregnancy may promote the growth of fibroids. Medications containing estrogen may also stimulate fibroid growth. When estrogen production naturally decreases during menopause, fibroids typically disappear. Also, fibroids tend to "run in the family."

TREATMENT OF FIBROIDS

Most women with fibroids require no treatment. The best course is what we call "watchful waiting," meaning that you don't do anything unless problems crop up or symptoms get worse. For women who do need treatment, here are the options:

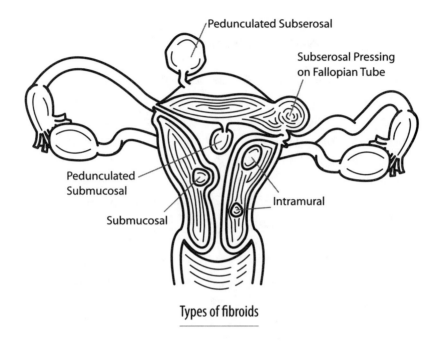

Types of fibroids

Medications

- Gonadotropin-releasing hormone agonists or GnRH (Lupron, Synarel). These are given by injection. They suppress the development of eggs and therefore the production of estrogen and progesterone. This puts you into temporary artificial menopause so that fibroids shrink just as they would with natural menopause. Your fertility will return within a few weeks after the treatment ends. During treatment you may have menopausal symptoms such as hot flashes.
- Testosterone (Danazol). This is a synthetic version of the male hormone, also called androgen. It stops your period and helps fibroids shrink but you may experience unpleasant side effects including growing facial and other unwanted hair and having your voice get lower. Also common are headaches, acne, and weight gain. (See chapter 2 for more information about testosterone/androgen treatments.)

One Woman's Story: Jillian, Age 31

"My husband and I really wanted kids. We started trying right after our first anniversary, but month after month I would still get my period. Finally almost a year later, the strip on the home test turned the right color. We were ecstatic! Then when the doctor did an ultrasound, she saw a huge fibroid. A couple of weeks later, I lost the baby. Awful, just awful! The doctor said the fibroid was so big that it had to come out. It probably took blood that should have gone to the baby. Also, I had been having really heavy periods for quite a while and a blood test showed that I was severely anemic. I had been having a lot of pain with my periods as well.

"We started talking about treatment options and the doctor asked me if I wanted to 'preserve my fertility.' Well, duh! Did he think I was going to let him do a hysterectomy? No way! What we decided on was that I would take medication to stop my periods so the fibroid would shrink. If it didn't totally shrink, at least they could get it out more easily during surgery. That sounded like a good plan at first, but just imagine how scary it is to have hot flashes and no periods when you're still hoping to start a family! The doctor assured me everything would go back to normal but I was crying all the time. The fibroid did get smaller, though, and after three months on the medication I had the procedure. I got pregnant six months later! Now we are the proud parents of the most beautiful baby girl in the world. Sure, more fibroids could grow down the line, but there was no way I was going to have a hysterectomy and miss out on being a mom."

Surgery

- Myomectomy. This procedure removes fibroids while leaving the uterus in place and preserving fertility. However, fibroids

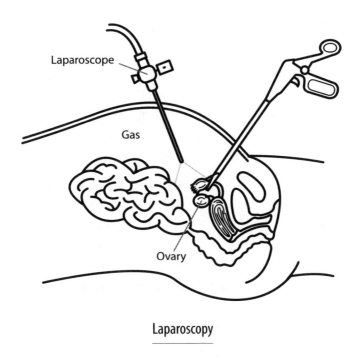

Laparoscopy

can recur after a myomectomy. For large fibroids, an abdominal incision may be necessary. Smaller fibroids can usually be removed with a laparoscopic procedure that requires only a tiny incision. Another possibility is a hysteroscopic procedure that allows your doctor to remove the fibroids vaginally. Variations of the hysteroscopic procedure include myolysis (an electric current to destroy the tumors) and cryomyolysis (freezing of the tumors).

- Endometrial ablation. This is a hysteroscopic procedure that uses heat to destroy the lining of the uterus. Most women are infertile after an ablation so it's not a good option if you want more children.
- Hysterectomy. Removal of the uterus is the only way to prevent the possibility of fibroids recurring, but you definitely won't be able to have children after a hysterectomy. (See "Hysterectomies," page 231.)

ENDOMETRIOSIS

This is a disorder in which the uterine lining, or endometrium, grows outside the uterus, most often on your fallopian tubes or ovaries. The tissue, called implants, bleeds every month just like your normal endometrium does, but the blood can't get out through your vagina. The result can be scar tissue, adhesions, and cysts that cause pain. Beyond that, endometriosis is a leading cause of infertility. For this reason, if you want to have more children, you should pay close attention to your health radar and ask for tests if you suspect you have endometriosis. As I like to say, be a "squeaky wheel"!

HOW TO TELL IF YOU HAVE ENDOMETRIOSIS

Endometriosis is a great masquerader. The symptoms are a lot like the symptoms of other problems "down there." I've had patients who thought they had inflammatory bowel disease or fibroids. Other patients, though, had no symptoms and the endometriosis wasn't discovered until they had laparoscopy or surgery for something else such as fibroids, infertility, or a tubal ligation.

Symptoms

- chronic pelvic pain
- painful periods
- heavy periods
- bleeding between periods
- bowel problems

Diagnostic Tests

- a pelvic exam with bimanual palpation (see chapter 3)
- Ultrasound. A diagnosis isn't possible unless cysts have formed. The actual implants are rarely visible.

- Laparoscopy. This procedure is the only one that gives a definitive diagnosis. (See "Fibroids," page 217.)

CAUSES OF ENDOMETRIOSIS

There are many theories but all we really know is that endometriosis runs in families. A genetic tendency to a hormone imbalance with lower than normal progesterone appears to be the reason, but nobody is sure about this.

TREATMENT OF ENDOMETRIOSIS

- Hormonal therapy. Birth controls pills and patches that result in lighter-than-normal periods can help reduce pain from endometriosis in mild cases. Other hormones that put you into artificial menopause can also be tried. (See "Fibroids," page 217, for a full explanation of these therapies.)

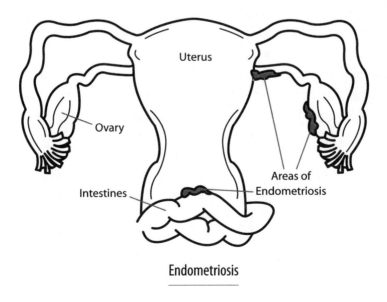

Endometriosis

PCOS (Polycystic Ovary Syndrome)

In 1935 seven women were reported with the combination of the following problems: amenorrhea (meaning no period, though anovulatory cycles with irregular periods are more typical), obesity (primarily belly fat and therefore an apple shape), hirsutism (abnormal hair growth in male pattern distribution), and a typical appearance on the ovaries of multiple cysts at surgery. (Ultrasound was not available back then). This report was published by two physicians, Drs. Stein and Levinthal. When I was in medical school, we called PCOS the "Stein-Levinthal syndrome," having not yet coined the confusing and not very helpful term "polycystic ovary syndrome."

Today the medically established criteria require that other causes of irregular periods and androgen "excess" or imbalance are ruled out or excluded and that two of the following are present: reduced or absent ovulation (infrequent/irregular or no periods at all), elevated levels of androgens or clinical signs of excess androgen regardless of blood test results (e.g., acne, hirsutism), and/or polycystic ovaries as seen on an ultrasound. In other words, ovaries and adrenal glands produce excess androgens in the form of testosterone, which lead to insulin resistance, ovarian cysts, and obesity, in particular belly fat and an apple shape.

Normally the ovaries produce androgens in response to pituitary LH (luteinizing hormone), which then gets converted to testosterone or estrogen. Women with PCOS are more efficient at producing testosterone than estrone, so the androgen/estrogen imbalance is at the heart of the problem. The ovaries normally produce more estrone in response to FSH (follicle-stimulating hormone) so with PCOS women have higher LH and therefore androgen production than they have FSH and estrone production. Insulin helps encourage androgen production by the ovaries, so higher insulin levels mean higher androgens. Insulin also reduces sex-binding protein so more testosterone is unbound and free to act on the body.

Women with PCOS are prone to increased metabolic and cardiovascular problems. This syndrome occurs in 5 to 10 percent of women. Since they don't ovulate regularly if at all, they have higher risk of endometrial lining buildup or hyperplasia and even cancer because they don't get the balancing progesterone during ovulation that would act to mature and then shed the uterine lining.

What to do if you have PCOS:

- Waist loss/weight loss: Even modest amounts of weight/waist loss is linked with improved ovulation. I would recommend working with a nutritionist before beginning medications for ovulation/insulin resistance.
- Oral contraceptives: The estrogen component suppresses or dampens the luteinizing hormone (LH). This in turn lowers androgen production and increases sex-binding proteins so there is less of the active testosterone circulating (see chapter 2). The progestin component helps to balance out the estrogen effect in the uterus and causes shedding and thinning of lining.
- Anti-androgens (androgen-blocking drugs): Spironolactone (a unique anti-adrenal mild diuretic used in women with premenstrual fluid retention and heart failure patients) blocks androgen if it is used in higher doses than normal (100 to 200 mg/day).
- Metformin (Glucophage): Used for diabetics as well, this medication helps with weight loss and helps to improve ovulation.
- Pioglitazone/Actos (and rosiglitazone/Avandia): Usually used for diabetics, these medications lower insulin and therefore androgen levels. They also promote weight gain but this is probably from fluid gain and not from visceral fat gain. An Avandia study did show improved ovulation. However, concerns about safety and pregnancy limits the use of these medications.

- Laparoscopy or abdominal surgery to remove the implants while leaving your reproductive organs intact.
- Assisted Reproductive Technology (ART) such as in vitro fertilization (IVF) may be helpful if endometriosis has caused infertility.
- Getting pregnant. In medical school I learned this is one way to get rid of the disease. I don't recommend getting pregnant just to treat endometriosis but if you want a baby anyway, this solution apparently works as well as anything else.
- Hysterectomy is a last resort. For severe cases of endometriosis, removal of the uterus ends the chronic pain but it also ends your fertility. (See page 231 for information about hysterectomies.)

PELVIC INFLAMMATORY DISEASE (PID)

As you learned back in chapter 2, STIs that are left untreated can spread to your internal reproductive organs. The resulting infections can cause pelvic inflammatory disease (PID), which in turn can lead to infertility or cause problems during pregnancy. Some cases are asymptomatic but if you do have symptoms, call your doctor to get help before damage is done.

HOW TO TELL IF YOU HAVE PID
Symptoms

- pelvic and lower abdominal pain
- fever
- vomiting
- heavy, foul-smelling vaginal discharge
- irregular periods
- difficulty urinating
- pain during sex

Diagnostic Tests

- a bimanual pelvic exam (see chapter 3)
- laboratory tests of samples of vaginal discharge and cervical tissue
- possibly an exploratory laparoscopic procedure to see how widespread the problem is (see "Fibroids," earlier in this chapter.)

CAUSES OF PID

- untreated gonorrhea (GC) or chlamydia (see chapter 2)
- bacterial infections that get into your vagina while your cervix is open such as during childbirth, miscarriage, abortion, or a procedure called endometrial biopsy
- bacteria acquired when you insert an intrauterine device (IUD) (see chapter 5, page 153)

TREATMENT OF PID

Oral antibiotics work well in most cases. Serious cases may require a hospital stay for intravenous antibiotics. If abscesses have formed, your doctor may recommend surgery to drain them but this is rare.

VULVODYNIA

This disorder is aptly named. The medical suffix "dynia" comes from the Greek word for pain. Women with vulvodynia report pain in the vulvar region that is often excruciating and almost always chronic. Vulvodynia was formerly called "vulvar vestibulitis," a term that meant "fear of penetration." (See chapter 1 for a description of the vestibule.) To me, that was off base. First of all, "itis" means "inflammation" and there is no inflammation associated with the disorder. Second, the term made it sound as though the afflicted woman was imagining the pain because she didn't want to have intercourse. I know from my experience with patients that the opposite is true. I remember feeling absolutely frustrated at times trying to help women who had chronic vulvar pain, not just with sex but with activities like bike riding or putting in a tampon. Yet when I was in medical school in the 1970s, the topic of vulvar pain was never mentioned. In fact, the first ever National Vulvodynia Awareness Campaign was launched in 2007 by the National Institutes of Health.

If you believe you have vulvodynia but your doctor doesn't know what you're talking about or seems to think it's all in your head, find a doctor who gets it! As a woman, I am empathetic. I really do feel my patients' pain. Fortunately for me, I never had a chronic problem but I will never forget the pain I experienced when my husband and I tried to have sex after my first son was born. I thought I was being torn apart. Over time the problem went away, but with my second pregnancy I was terrified that it would come back again. It didn't, but I can definitely sympathize with my patients who report chronic vulvar pain.

No one knows what causes vulvodynia. There are no tests available to diagnose the disorder, but your doctor may do tests to rule out other disorders that cause pain and itching such as vaginitis.

SYMPTOMS OF VULVODYNIA

- pain with sex or when inserting anything such as a diaphragm or a tampon into the vagina
- pain with contact to the vulva such as when bike riding, horseback riding, or even sitting for long periods or wearing tight jeans
- constant or intermittent vulvar pain for no discernible reason (patients variously describe the pain as burning, itching, stinging, and throbbing).

TREATMENT OF VULVODYNIA
Medications

- Anticonvulsants such as Tegretol and Neurontin sometimes ease the symptoms.

- Tricyclic antidepressants (Norpramin, Elavil) may help.
- Antihistamines can lessen pain and reduce itching.
- Physical Therapy

Your doctor may give you a prescription for physical therapy to strengthen pelvic floor muscles.

Topical Anesthetic
A cream such as Lidocaine may help numb the pain during sex. Your partner will end up feeling numb for a while as well.

Cold Compresses
This is an age-old home remedy that does relieve pain temporarily.

GYNECOLOGIC CANCERS

Some cancers can be hereditary. If your female relatives had cancer of any organ of the reproductive tract at an early age, let your doctor know. For example, if your mother or a close female relative had ovarian cancer in her forties, you can be screened for that disease even though the test is not routinely performed. The earlier the cancer is detected, the better the prognosis.

The most common types of cancers of the female reproductive organs are cervical, vulvar, vaginal, endometrial, and ovarian. Cancer of the fallopian tubes is rare. Rarer still is a type of cancer that develops during conception or at the site of the placenta after delivery of a baby.

CAUSES AND PREVENTION
We don't know what causes most forms of gynecologic cancer but we do know that the human papillomavirus (HPV) causes cervical cancer. HPV can also cause vulvar, vaginal, oral, and anal cancers, and rare penile cancers in men, too. The good news is that in addition to the Pap

smear, we now have a test for HPV as well as a vaccine (see chapter 2 for complete information).

SYMPTOMS AND TESTS

In the earliest stages, most cancers are asymptomatic. Also, any symptoms you do experience are similar to those for less serious problems: heavy, painful, or irregular periods; pelvic pain; low back pain; and vaginal discharge. This is why you should never ignore symptoms even if they're not all that bothersome. Pay attention to your health radar and call your doctor whenever you sense that something is off-kilter. Many of the exams and tests I've described for other disorders, including a routine pelvic exam, can lead to detection of cancer or lead your doctor to do further testing if cancer is suspected.

TREATMENT OF CANCER

Depending on the type and stage of cancer, treatment can include chemotherapy, radiation, and surgery. Sometimes the diseased area can be

Is There a Screening Test for Ovarian Cancer?

Although there is no surefire screening test for ovarian cancer, researchers are working on finding a way to detect this disease. For now, the best we have is the annual pelvic exam but early ovarian cancer is often missed. However, if you have any combination of the following symptoms for two to three weeks, your doctor can do an ultrasound and order a blood test to check for a tumor marker called Cancer Antigen 125 (CA-125).

- a feeling of being full even though you haven't eaten much
- bloating
- pelvic pain
- frequent need to urinate

removed or destroyed while leaving the rest of your reproductive organs intact (see chapter 2, page 51). In advanced cases, a hysterectomy may be the best treatment option. However, even then you may not need a hysterectomy that removes all of your reproductive organs. In the next section, I'll tell you about the types of hysterectomies that are available.

HYSTERECTOMIES

I remember not so long ago when insurance companies started requiring a "second opinion" for certain procedures, including hysterectomies. Before then, most patients wouldn't risk offending their primary physicians by telling them that they wanted a second opinion. I must confess that many years ago I did feel a bit threatened if a patient asked for advice about which doctor to see for another opinion. Yet for the thousands of women who were having unnecessary hysterectomies, getting a second opinion suddenly seemed to me to be a great way to protect women from overly aggressive surgeons.

True, a hysterectomy is sometimes the best option. However, the widespread practice of removing perfectly healthy ovaries at the time of surgery "just in case" had always given me great concern. This custom among surgeons seems to presume that after menopause the ovaries are nothing more than spare parts. Yet even when we no longer have eggs available for fertilization, our ovaries remain hormone powerhouses to a degree that is not yet fully understood. Some doctors feel that all you need to do if the ovaries are removed is to take estrogen replacement therapy. Wrong! As you learned in chapter 2, not only estrogen but also testosterone is vital for maintaining our sense of well-being, libido, and muscle strength. Yet testosterone replacement for women is no easy or straightforward matter. Beyond all that, removing the ovaries is no guarantee that you won't get cancer. Ovarian cancer does not always arise from the ovaries but from primitive cells throughout the peritoneal cavity. These cells can't be identified and removed until they have already developed into cancer. Even prophylactic ovary removal in women who inherit BRCA 1 or 2 genes (see chapter 3) does not completely protect them from future ovarian cancer.

Here is something else you may not have thought about. Should you have your perfectly healthy cervix removed along with your uterus during a hysterectomy? You're not going to get pregnant after a hysterectomy anyway, so you may wonder why you would want to keep the organ that needs regular scraping for a Pap test and that could develop cervical cancer. The reason is that the cervix is thought to play a role in sexual pleasure.

Now here is one of the best-kept secrets: Always look for a surgeon who does minimally invasive hysterectomies—either vaginally, robotically, or laparoscopically. If your doctor isn't trained in the newer techniques, he may not tell you about these options. Up to one-half of all hysterectomies are still done with an abdominal incision. In some cases that may be necessary but not many. Speak up!

With all of that in mind, here are the different types of hysterectomies:

- Partial or subtotal. This procedure removes the uterus but leaves the cervix, ovaries, and fallopian tubes in place.
- Complete or total. These terms are misleading. They refer to a procedure that removes the uterus and the cervix but not the ovaries and the fallopian tubes.
- Radical. This procedure removes the uterus, the upper part of the vagina, the cervix, supporting tissues, one or both ovaries, and the fallopian tubes.

If you have advanced cancer, then a radical hysterectomy that could remove all of the diseased tissues may well be a good choice. But if you have fibroids, chronic pelvic pain, endometriosis, or the early stages of gynecologic cancers, please get a second or even a third opinion regarding the need for a hysterectomy, radical or not. If a conservative

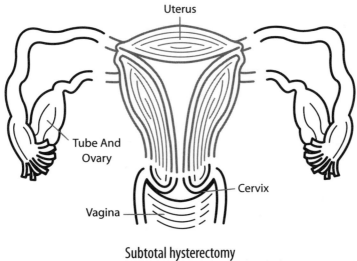

Subtotal hysterectomy

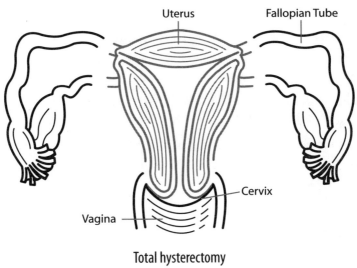

Total hysterectomy

treatment turns out to be a prudent option—and perhaps a minimally invasive procedure rather than open laparotomy, which takes weeks of recovery rather than days—you'll be very glad you stayed in control of your own health care.

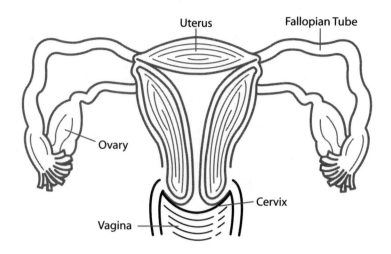

Bilateral salpingo-oophorectomy (ovaries removed)

This chapter was all about the parts that only women have. The next chapter, though, underscores my point that even when it comes to other organs, women are not just "small men." We have a much slower digestive process than men do so we are three times more likely to experience bowel problems. Fortunately, simple lifestyle changes can help you cope with most of these. I'll tell you what you need to know in order to keep everything moving the way it should.

8

Internal Plumbing Down There

Bowel Problems from Cause to Cure

IN THIS CHAPTER

- How Your Bowels Are Supposed to Work

- Constipation

- Hemorrhoids

- Irritable Bowel Syndrome (IBS)

- Diarrhea

Based on my quarter century as a practicing physician, I'm convinced that just about everybody has to deal with at least one bowel issue at some point. A now classic study done at the University of North Carolina in 1993 showed that 69 percent of the participants had experienced one or more gastrointestinal disorders in the previous three months. The research also showed that people with these disorders were more inclined to absenteeism, or taking sick days, than were the other participants. What's more, a 2004 article in the *Harvard Business Review* listed gastrointestinal disorders as one of the leading causes of a phenomenon dubbed "presenteeism" in which people report to work but don't get much done. Obviously, a regular bowel movement is important!

As for me, I never thought much about my intestinal tract until after my first son was born. Except for an attack of Montezuma's revenge that had me doubled over in pain and running to the bathroom with diarrhea during a vacation in Mexico, my bowels functioned fine. When I gave birth, however, I ended up with what I was sure was the biggest hemorrhoid ever. Having a bowel movement was incredibly painful. That experience helped me to understand what my patients with bowel complaints had been going through over the years. Bowel problems, whether they're minor or major, not only typically make you miserable but they are also something most of us feel uncomfortable discussing. Yet they are in general fairly easy to avoid and treat, often with home remedies and a few lifestyle changes. Also, the most serious problem—colon cancer—is preventable. My goal in this chapter is to give you all the information you need in order to have a healthy digestive system and to cope well with any upsets you do encounter.

HOW YOUR BOWELS ARE SUPPOSED TO WORK

The small intestine connects to the colon, or large intestine, which is almost five feet long. It fits easily into your abdominal cavity because it's coiled back and forth like a garden hose. At the bottom end it connects to the rectum and the anus (see chapter 1 for definitions of these terms). The major function of the colon is to store waste materials from the food you eat. About two pints of liquid matter enter the colon from the small intestine each day. The colon absorbs water, nutrients, and salts from that liquid. What's left, the stool, is about a third of a pint.

PERISTALSIS

The rhythmic contractions of the muscles of the colon that push the stool through the colon are part of a process called peristalsis. It begins in your esophagus after you swallow food and continues until you have a bowel movement. Peristalsis is regulated by nerves and hormones working together to send messages from the brain to the gastrointestinal tract. If the muscles of the colon and the anal sphincters ("pinch tight muscles") don't contract and relax correctly, the contents of the colon don't move as they should. I'll teach you about the symptoms and disorders that result when that happens. Let's start with the most common complaint, constipation.

CONSTIPATION

The frequency of bowel movements varies widely. Some medical textbooks teach that any pattern is "normal" if it's your usual one. However, I believe that what is "normal" for you and what would be optimal functioning for your colon can be two different scenarios. Some people go once or twice a day, others once every two or three days. The latter pattern can be classified as "normal," but there's no getting around the fact that the longer stool sits in the colon, the more compact and dense it becomes. This makes having a bowel movement more difficult, which can lead to other problems as well. If you typically don't have a bowel movement every day, study this section so that you can decide whether simple changes might alter your bowel habits for the better. Women have much slower intestinal peristalsis than men and as a result are at least three times more vulnerable to chronic constipation. The good news, however, is that preventing and treating constipation is something you can almost always do on your own, usually without a trip to the doctor or the need for prescription medication.

SYMPTOMS OF CONSTIPATION

Bowel movement infrequency is only one component of chronic constipation. According to several large epidemiologic studies, patients with chronic constipation report straining, a sense of incomplete or ineffective defecation, and hard or lumpy stools as the most bothersome symptoms of constipation. According to a standard set of criteria, a patient is constipated if she has at least two of the following symptoms present for at least three months:

- hard stools
- straining while trying to pass stools
- sensation of incomplete emptying or evacuation at least 25 percent of the time
- two or fewer bowel movements per week

What Is Safe Toilet Syndrome?

A phenomenon called the "safe toilet syndrome" happens when people "hold it in" until they get home from a prolonged business trip or vacation because they don't feel comfortable going in a strange place. This can also happen when people are hospitalized. There's nothing like sharing a toilet with a very sick roommate to make a person want to avoid bowel movements!

In truth, though, no one needs a set of criteria. You *know* when you're constipated and the "knowing" may be different for each of us. This is a perfect example of my often-stated fact: You know when your body is not right. Your health radar works better for you than any objective diagnosis. Believe it.

WHEN TO SEE A DOCTOR FOR CONSTIPATION

Most people with constipation don't need to undergo testing. However, if you experience any of the following red flags for colon cancer, make an appointment to see your doctor:

- unexpected weight loss
- sudden change in bowel habits
- blood in the stool—visible or hidden (occult)—that is not from hemorrhoids (see chapter 3 and "Hemorrhoids," page 246)

CAUSES OF CONSTIPATION

- Not eating enough fiber. Fiber provides the bulk that helps to speed the passage of waste through the bowel. Without enough fiber, stools are harder, more compact, and take longer to move through the colon. I think of the colon as a muscle that needs a daily workout. The best workout involves lots of fiber that stretches the muscle, then a good evacuation where the muscle gets to spring back into place. If chronic constipation causes the colon to stretch beyond a certain point, it loses its elasticity so that it no longer bounces back. Think of a shower cap with stretched out elastic that doesn't fit snugly.

- Not drinking enough fluids. The body needs one and a half to two quarts a day to function efficiently. Without sufficient fluids, waste matter in the colon becomes too hard, making passage through the bowel more difficult.

- Not enough physical activity. This may be the single most important factor that causes constipation. It's a huge problem especially for the elderly and for people confined to bed or wheelchairs. It's also an issue for people who take long airplane, train, or car rides or simply sit working at desks all day. If you don't stay physically active, your entire system slows down, including the muscle contractions that move waste matter through the bowel.

- Ignoring the need to go because you're too busy. Women with small children often fall prey to this problem, especially if the

Do Coffee, Tea, and Sodas Count as Fluid Intake?

Fluids other than water do count toward your daily quota. Coffee in moderation, even decaffeinated coffee, is a stimulant that can trigger your morning bowel movement. Tea, on the other hand, contains tannin that may slow down peristalsis. As for sodas, both the regular and so-called "diet" versions are poor choices. The refined sugar in regular sodas gives you "empty calories" and the artificial sweeteners in the "diet" sodas can actually make you fat!

One Woman's Story: Lois, Age 57

"I'm a voice teacher in the city but one summer I had the opportunity to join the faculty of a fine arts summer camp in a gorgeous mountain setting by a lake. My kids are grown and I'm divorced so that seemed like a chance to relive my own wonderful experiences as a camper. Well! Being on the adult side of the equation was a whole 'nother thing! I've never been so busy in my life—not even when my three children were little.

"The faculty was pretty much on call 24/7 not just to teach but also to supervise meals and bedtime and to rehearse for the final concert. Besides that, I was living in a cabin with three other teachers and one bathroom for all four of us. By week three, I realized I hadn't had a bowel movement in five days! I just never had time to go when I felt the urge. I was so uncomfortable! No amount of straining did any good. I hated the idea of starting to take anything because my grandmother had been the laxative queen. I've never forgotten that. She talked about it all the time and she was also always giving herself enemas. What I did was walk into the nearby town on my day off and buy a big box of All-Bran. I felt a little more bloated at first from the extra fiber but by week's end it had worked like a charm.

"To this day, I eat All-Bran every single morning plus lots of fresh fruits and veggies and I drink plenty of water. I've never been constipated since that one episode. Fiber does it for me!"

children want to come into the bathroom with you as my three boys always did!

- "Holiday constipation" when any change of routine or diet can cause problems with the digestive tract.
- Pregnancy. The increase in the hormone progesterone tends to slow down contractions of the colon. That, along with

the weight and size of the pregnant uterus, contributes to
constipation during pregnancy.

- large uterine fibroids (see chapter 7, page 217)
- prescription medications, particularly antidepressants,
  narcotic-like painkillers, water pills (diuretics), and the
  calcium channel blocker verapamil used to treat high blood
  pressure and angina
- over-the-counter medicines including antihistamines (Benadryl),
  cough medicines (with Phenergan or codeine), and drugs used
  to treat diarrhea (Imodium, Lomotil), antacids containing
  aluminum, and iron tablets (even the 18 mg of iron in a
  multivitamin can do it for some women)
- An underactive thyroid gland (hypothyroidism). This metabolic
  disorder leads to reduced peristalsis.
- nerve damage in the gastrointestinal tract caused by underlying
  conditions such as diabetes and multiple sclerosis
- psychological problems, including depression
- bowel disorders that make going to the bathroom painful—
  anything from hemorrhoids and small tears or fissures to colon
  cancer
- Diverticular disease. Many people over forty develop bulging
  pouches in the large intestive called diverticula. The condition
  is called diverticulosis. If the diverticula become inflamed
  or infected, the condition is called diverticulitis. Symptoms
  include abdominal pain, nausea, and constipation. A recent
  study debunked the long-held myth that eating nuts, corn, and
  popcorn aggravates the problem. In fact these foods along with
  other high fiber choices help prevent diverticular disease.

TREATMENT FOR CONSTIPATION

Along with drinking plenty of fluids and leading an active lifestyle, a diet
rich in fiber is your best defense against constipation. Plants—meaning

What Causes Bloating?

When you're constipated, the bacteria that live in your colon use the undigested sugars in the compacted waste products for fuel. That process produces gas. Other causes of bloating are spastic colon, or irritable bowel syndrome (see the section on IBS later in this chapter) and lactose intolerance in which the undigested or partially digested milk sugar, lactose, is fermented by bowel bacteria. Artificial sweeteners with sorbitol in sugar-free candies and gum can also cause gas. I once thought I had acute appendicitis after I ate a whole bag of sugar-free gummies! Also, the chewable fiber supplement sold as Benefiber contains artificial sweeteners that can lead to gas.

fruits (especially prunes), vegetables, and grains—are the only natural source of fiber. As a rule of thumb, eat fresh produce rather than processed food that is typically stripped not only of fiber content but of vitamins and other nutrients as well. In other words, an apple is a better choice than apple juice or apple sauce.

The following foods are all good sources of dietary fiber:

- beans, lentils, and peas
- fresh and dried fruits—particularly if you eat the skins
- vegetables—particularly if you eat the skins
- nuts and seeds
- whole-grain breads
- skin of potatoes
- whole-grain breakfast cereals
- whole-grain pasta
- brown rice

Dietary Fiber Supplements

These supplements do improve stool frequency and consistency, but they don't come with the phytonutrients and antioxidants in high-fiber foods that help protect against cancer and also slow the effects of aging.

I remember that there was only one fiber supplement available when I felt I needed one after my son was born in 1980. It was the original gray-white, non-flavored Metamucil in powder form that had to be mixed with juice or water. I learned to drink it down quickly before it turned into a gooey blob. Today there are many choices including Metamucil's "Berry Burst" formula that is promoted with cheery advertising copy: "Berry Beautiful Bowels—a tasteful way to doll up digestion and help lower your cholesterol so your heart can look irresistible. Metamucil. Beautify your inside."

Here's what you can buy over the counter at your grocery store or drugstore:

Natural Fiber Supplements

- psyllium (Metamucil)
- wheat dextrin (Benefiber) (see above for information on bloating)

Dr. Marie's Four "F" Prescription for Preventing Constipation:

Fitness, Fluids, Fiber, and Frequency

What I mean is that you need to stay physically active, drink plenty of fluids every day, eat a diet high in natural fibers from plants, and go when you get the urge to go instead of "holding it in"!

What Are Stool Softeners?

Stool softeners are "add-ons" for the bowel regimens of patients with chronic pain from hemorrhoids as well as patients on narcotics that bring colon motility to an abrupt stop. One brand name is Colace. Peri-Colace is a combination product that works as a softener and also has senna, the same ingredient in Ex-Lax.

Synthetic Fiber Supplement

- calcium polycarbophil (FiberCon)

Osmotic Laxatives

Osmotic laxatives keep more fluid than normal in the colon so that the stool is more liquid than usual and thus more easily passed. Here are the types:

- Magnesium (milk of magnesia). This product has been a bestseller since 1880!
- polyethylene glycol (Miralax)
- polyethylene glycol with electrolytes (Golytely and Colyte.

Is Mineral Oil a Safe Laxative?

No! Mineral oil can be aspirated into the lungs. The oil, which acts more as a stool softener than as a laxative, was commonly taken in the past to ease the passage of stools, but the practice is now considered dangerous.

These are used to clean out the colon before a colonoscopy. You need a prescription.)

- synthetic sugars (Sorbitol and lactulose. One brand name is Chronulac. You need a prescription. Bloating is a common side effect. The artificial sugars taste sweet but are not metabolized so they have no calories. They are also among the ingredients in sugar-free candies and gum.)

Suppositories and Enemas

Glycerin suppositories have an osmotic effect and were used regularly in my grandparents' day. Enemas were also used often. These choices are much less popular today. They do clean out the colon but they lack any of the nutrient benefits of a high-fiber diet and they don't promote good muscle tone in the colon.

Stimulant Laxatives

I remember that the most popular laxative I dispensed as a student nurse in the late 1960s was dubbed "chocolate and white" because it was a

Are the New Prescription Medications for Constipation Safe?

Only time will tell. Why be a guinea pig? In 2006 the FDA approved Amitiza (lubiprostone), which is now widely advertised. I have a feeling that the direct-to-consumer advertising budget far exceeds the research budget for this drug. As for Tegaserod, it is available for women under age fifty-five who have no cardiovascular risk factors and who have tried and failed other treatments for constipation. However, in 2007 studies showed that this drug increases cardiovascular events. It is no longer approved for use by older women or those with risk factors for heart disease.

Bulimia Nervosa and Addiction to Laxatives

People with the eating disorder called bulimia nervosa force themselves to vomit and also regularly use laxatives. Both of these practices are dangerous and can have long-term adverse effects on the colon. For that matter, anyone who becomes dependent on laxatives risks compromising the natural strength and elasticity of the colon. If you have symptoms of bulimia or feel that you may be addicted to laxatives, please get medical help right away.

combination of brown senna (Ex-Lax) along with white milk of magnesia. However, my physician husband recalls that "black and white" referred to the nursing remedy of prune juice and milk of magnesia. That version was probably safer. I was trained that stimulant laxatives such as Ex-Lax are potentially addictive and can be harmful if used long-term. Colon experts say these claims have never been substantiated but my personal experience has been that people who use stimulant laxatives often do not make lifestyle changes such as eating a high-fiber diet, drinking plenty of fluids, and getting enough exercise. They depend on the stimulant laxative effect alone to remain "regular." Here's the list of laxatives available. Use with caution, use sparingly, and use only as a last resort!

- senna (Ex-Lax)
- castor oil
- diphenylmethane (bisacodyl)

HEMORRHOIDS

As I mentioned earlier, when I gave birth for the first time, I ended up with a giant hemorrhoid that made having a bowel movement incredibly painful. I was barely able to enjoy the wonders of a new baby because I was so preoccupied with my sore bottom. On the plus side, though, I credit that episode with my devotion to eating well, including having plenty of fiber in my diet. I learned other ways to avoid and treat hemorrhoids as well. Since an estimated 90 percent of us will have at least one episode of hemorrhoids, also called piles, read on even if you're still among the fortunate few who haven't yet succumbed.

Technically, hemorrhoids are simply the veins in the rectum. However, the term is popularly used to refer to those veins when they have become inflamed and swollen with excess blood. They are varicose veins just like the ones you might get in your legs. I have found that people tend to think of hemorrhoids as something they catch rather than as just a swelling of normal anal tissue. Learning exactly what this tissue is and how it works will help you understand causes and cures for the inflammation.

The anal opening is also known as the anal verge. About an inch above this area is an important landmark known as the dentate line. It contains a circle of glands that secrete mucus that lubricates the anal canal to make the passage of stool easier. Surrounding this area there is a complex array of blood vessels, connective tissue, and smooth muscle that provides sensory information to our brains. That's how we get signals when we need to pass gas or have a bowel movement.

What Is Thrombosis?

Occasionally a blood vessel in the hemorrhoid tissue will form a clot called a thrombosis. The pain associated with this can be severe and the dread you will feel thinking about having a bowel movement is a major problem. See a doctor if you suspect you have this condition.

Should I Go to the Doctor If I See Blood in My Stool?

Yes, unless the cause is obviously a hemorrhoid and the symptom goes away when you follow my treatment tips. Never assume that persistent rectal bleeding is a minor problem that will disappear on its own. Rather, view it as a cause for alarm that requires a doctor's appointment so you can be screened for colon cancer. This is especially true if you are over the age of fifty, have a family history of colon cancer or a personal history of any cancer, have abdominal discomfort or pain, have altered bowel habits, or are experiencing unexplained weight loss.

Also, other than cancer, you may have a serious condition such as fissures or tears in the anal tissues, abscesses, or infections. Best case scenario, you'll turn out to have nothing more than an anal irritation caused by allergies to perfumed hygiene products or incomplete cleansing following a bowel movement. (Baby wipes to the rescue! See chapter 2.) But at least you'll have peace of mind when you find that out. Never feel foolish about going to the doctor when you have a scary symptom. She's hoping it's a false alarm just as much as you are! A final word: I hope you'll follow my advice about colon cancer screening in chapter 3. The earlier the cancer or precancerous condition is detected, the better the prognosis!

Enlarged veins below the dentate line are external hemorrhoids. When they first occur, you may feel nothing more than small swellings referred to by doctors as "skin tags." If they get bigger, they'll cause itching, burning, and pain. There are also veins above the dentate line. They can enlarge and become internal hemorrhoids. The veins above the line don't have nerve fibers, so internal hemorrhoids don't cause pain. However, they may pop out below the dentate line and protrude from the anal opening after a bowel movement. I have had many a worried patient come to me complaining about "something horrible sticking out" or "a growth." Others have even used the word "tumor."

SYMPTOMS OF HEMORRHOIDS

- swollen veins that protrude through the rectum, especially after you have strained to have a bowel movement
- blood in the stool or in the toilet bowl after a bowel movement (*Warning:* Blood in the stool, especially if the symptom persists, may be a sign of colon cancer or other problems. See the sidebar on page 248.)
- rectal discomfort including itching, burning, and pain

CAUSES OF HEMORRHOIDS

- Not enough fiber. A low-fiber diet leads to hard stools that are difficult to pass.
- Sitting too long on the toilet. You're putting pressure on the circular area of the buttocks while your rectal tissues are relaxed. I think of it as if you are applying a tourniquet to your pelvic area and allowing your delicate anal tissues below the tourniquet to bulge.
- Genetics. There is no concrete evidence that hemorrhoids run in the family but body shape does seem to play a part. Pear-shaped women who have hips that are proportionately larger than their waists tend to have hemorrhoids as well as varicose veins in their legs.
- Standing for too long. This is what triggers a flare-up of hemorrhoids for me. I always attend a string of holiday cocktail parties, so like clockwork I used to get hemorrhoids once a year. Now I make a point of finding a place to sit down every once in a while during the festivities!

Can I Get Hemorrhoids from Sitting on Cold Surfaces?

No, although sitting for long periods on cold surfaces such as a bench at a football game or a curb to watch a parade can make symptoms worse if you already have hemorrhoids. At first the low temperature will shrink the swollen veins but eventually your body will react by sending blood to warm your bottom. That makes your veins fill up even more than before. My mother, who was a nurse, always warned me not to sit on cold surfaces. As a little girl, I privately thought this advice was crazy. I later learned that mom was right after all! Of course, sitting on any hard surface, cold or not, isn't a good idea for more than a little while.

- Sitting for too long. This had been dubbed "truck driver's syndrome." It can happen as a result of long car or train rides and also when you sit at a desk for hours on end.
- Lifting heavy objects. Some people find that this makes the rectal veins pop out.

TREATMENT FOR HEMORRHOIDS
Lifestyle Changes

- a high-fiber diet rich in whole grains, fruits, and vegetables
- plenty of liquids
- an active lifestyle without long periods of standing still or sitting
- Breaking the habit of reading on the toilet. Just do your business as soon as you feel the urge and then get up!

Home Remedies and Over-the-Counter Treatments

- Gently push a hemorrhoid back in so that it can heal. Use a soapy finger in the shower or coat your finger with petroleum jelly.
- Apply ice packs. Put crushed ice cubes in a zippered plastic bag, wrap with a soft cloth, and apply the pack for about fifteen minutes while lying on your side. Don't sit on the pack and don't leave it on longer than recommended. (See the sidebar about cold surfaces, page 250.)
- Apply witch hazel. This liquid astringent has been used for generations to shrink hemorrhoids. (It can also safely tighten and smooth the skin on your face!) You can now buy towelettes moistened with witch hazel to carry with you. When I was a nurse in the 1960s on the postpartum floors, we used iced witch

Should I Use Preparation H?

I don't recommend using this over-the-counter product although it's been around since 1935. The active ingredient, phenylephrine, constricts blood vessels but the effect is temporary. In other words, Preparation H does not "cure" hemorrhoids and it certainly doesn't prevent them. It simply masks the symptoms for a while. You're better off with lifestyle changes and pain-relieving tactics.

On another note, do not use Preparation H for "off-label" purposes such as shrinking the bags under your eyes or toning "love handles." This alarming practice became fashionable in 2008 when word spread that models and body builders rely on the cream as a quick fix. However, many people end up with a scaly, eczema-like rash. Worse yet, applying Preparation H over relatively large areas of your skin can raise your blood pressure.

hazel compresses to give new mothers relief from hemorrhoids. I suspect this wonderful hands-on treatment may still be used today if the nurses have time for it. You can make a compress at home by soaking a soft cotton cloth with witch hazel and chilling it in the refrigerator. Use it for about fifteen minutes at a time.

- Apply petroleum jelly, cocoa butter, lanolin, mineral oil, glycerin, or a healing ointment called Aquaphor to relieve irritation and protect the inflamed tissues. Use after each bowel movement, making sure you cleanse first with nonallergenic baby wipes (see chapter 7).
- Apply topical hydrocortisone cream. This can relieve itching.
- Apply or insert topical anesthetics. Many products are available over the counter including Lanacane and Fleet Pain Relief. Use only according to the directions.
- Use Proctofoam-HC. You need a prescription for this pain-relieving foam that comes in a spray canister. I love this product!
- Sit on a donut cushion. These foam chair pads have a hole in the center so that you are putting less pressure on your anal area. They're available through pharmaceutical catalogs and at medical supply houses.
- Use fiber supplements and stool softeners to soften stools (see "Constipation," earlier in this chapter).

Office Procedures

If topical remedies don't work, a rectal specialist may treat you with one or more of the following:

- rubber band ligation, a very common procedure in which the doctor wraps a tiny rubber band around the base of each internal hemorrhoid to cut off blood supply
- sclerotherapy, an injection of a chemical solution to shrink the swollen tissues

Is a Sitz Bath a Good Idea When I Have Hemorrhoids?

No. A warm sitz bath probably does more harm than good. You'll be sitting on a rigid plastic basin that fits over the toilet. Only your buttocks will be in the water. This position can cause blood vessels to become congested, which only aggravates the problem. A sitz bath is an age-old remedy that many people still recommend but I don't agree! Reclining in a bathtub of warm water makes more sense, but who has time for that?

- coagulation therapy that uses lasers, infrared light, or radio waves to cut off circulation to the swollen veins
- cryotherapy that uses a liquid nitrogen probe inserted with an anoscope to freeze the tissues
- surgical hemorrhoidectomy, a procedure that is reserved for the most severe hemorrhoid cases and is much less frequently done today than it was years ago

IRRITABLE BOWEL SYNDROME (IBS)

While I was in private practice, I had a stack of hand-outs ready to give to my patients on various conditions. The most popular one by far was an article on IBS that I had written for *Woman's Day* magazine. As many as 20 percent of adults experience symptoms of IBS and 70 percent of people with IBS are women. The syndrome begins before the age of thirty-five in about 50 percent of people who have it.

The famous Canadian physician Sir William Osler coined the term "mucous colitis" in 1892 when he wrote of a disorder characterized by "mucorrhea and abdominal colic." Since that time, the syndrome has been referred to by many terms including spastic colon and nervous colon. For the sake of clarity, I'm going to use irritable bowel syndrome or IBS throughout this section.

IBS is what doctors call a "diagnosis of exclusion." We rule out other possibilities based on the fact that there is no blood in the stool; no family history of colon cancer or inflammatory bowel disease (see sidebar on page 255); no abdominal masses; and negative results on a group of tests including a colonoscopy and blood work for thyroid disorder.

IBS is a chronic, recurring gastro-intestinal problem. Although IBS does not lead to serious diseases, it can make your life miserable. The good news, though, is that you can learn to manage your symptoms and live well with this condition.

SYMPTOMS OF IBS

People with IBS sometimes alternate among symptoms. Certain patients find that their symptoms subside for a few months and then return while others report a gradual worsening of symptoms over time.

- abdominal pain that is relieved by having a bowel movement
- frequent bloating
- a change in the appearance or frequency of stools
- mucus in stools
- constipation
- cramping when trying to have a bowel movement
- diarrhea with an urgent need to get to the bathroom before it's too late

DIAGNOSTIC TESTS FOR IBS

There is no specific test for IBS although your doctor will perform tests to make sure you don't have other problems. These tests typically include:

- stool samples to look for hidden blood, parasites, and infections

Is IBS the Same as IBD?

No! Irritable bowel syndrome (IBS) should not be confused with inflammatory bowel disease (IBD). The latter term refers to two serious disorders, Crohn's disease and ulcerative colitis. A third serious disease that affects the digestive system is called celiac. All three of these problems most often affect people in their teens and twenties although they can occur later as well. The symptoms are similar to those for other bowel problems but they are typically more persistent and severe. If you think you might have IBD or celiac disease, see a doctor for an examination and tests.

- complete blood tests including thyroid function and something called "sedimentation rate," which checks for systemic inflammation
- gastrointestinal tests such as an upper endoscopy to check the upper GI tract for problems and a colonoscopy to check the colon, primarily if you are over fifty or have other risk factors for colon cancer or inflammatory bowel disease

If all your tests are negative, your doctor will make the diagnosis of IBS based on your symptoms. This is one time your health journal (see chapter 3) will really come in handy! Your doctor will want to know:

- how often you have had abdominal pain or discomfort during the past year
- when the pain starts and stops in relation to bowel function
- whether your bowel frequency and stool consistency have changed
- whether you have more symptoms during your period, since research has suggested that hormones may play a role

CAUSES OF IBS

Researchers have yet to discover any specific cause for IBS. Everything from stress to diet to allergies to an altered immune system has been studied with no conclusive results. There was a time during the early years of my practice when we tested patients' stools for a parasite called giardia as well as for other parasites. Whether or not we found any "bugs," we prescribed the antibiotic Flagyl. It didn't work.

The most recent theory is that serotonin, the hormone that plays a part in depression and migraines when people don't have enough of it, may cause IBS when there is too much of it. Ninety-five percent of the serotonin in your body is located in the GI tract. The other 5 percent is in the brain. Serotonin is a chemical that delivers messages or "mail" from one part of your body to another. Cells that line the inside of the bowel work as mail carriers. They carry the serotonin out of the GI tract. People with IBS may have faulty messengers that leave abnormally high levels of serotonin in the GI tract. This could be what causes bowel problems and abdominal pain but we don't know for sure. However, since our bowels require such a complex and sophisticated interplay of activities in order to work properly, the prevalence of IBS

What Are Probiotics?

According to the November 1, 2008, issue of *American Family Physician,* probiotics—live cultures of the genus of bacteria called lactobacillus—can help improve immune function, restore a healthy balance of bowel bacteria, and reduce symptoms of IBS. More and more products are appearing on grocery shelves. Probiotics are apparently stimulated by soluble dietary fiber so they are more likely to proliferate in the colon if you eat them along with legumes, veggies, and grains.

should come as no surprise. Any number of insults, disturbances, and imbalances in the system could upset normal functioning even if we haven't yet pinpointed what those might be.

TREATMENT FOR IBS

Lifestyle Changes

The information regarding constipation earlier in this chapter applies to IBS as well. In particular, remember my four Fs: fitness, fluids, fiber, and frequency. Beyond that, eat slowly so you won't swallow air that can cause belching and gas. For the same reason, don't chew gum. Also, avoid large meals that can cause bloating, cramping, and diarrhea.

In addition, keep a food diary to learn what triggers your symptoms. Common culprits include:

- caffeine
- corn
- dairy products containing lactose
- wheat products
- beans
- broccoli
- sugar-free candies and gum containing sorbitol
- carbonated beverages

Medications

Medication can sometimes relieve the symptoms of IBS, at least temporarily, but I recommend trying lifestyle changes first. The medications include:

Medications for Spasm

Muscle relaxants slow down contractions of the colon but they have side effects similar to Benadryl and other antihistamines including sleepiness, fatigue, and a general "cloudy" feeling. They can also make

What is Bowel Incontinence?

Any time you can't hold a bowel movement in, such as during a bout of acute diarrhea, is an episode of bowel incontinence. However, for some people the condition, also called fecal incontinence, is chronic. One cause is nerve damage sustained during childbirth and another is weakening of the anal sphincters ("pinch tight" muscles) due to aging.

However, the most common cause of stool accidents, whether occasional leaks or total loss of control, is a routine episiotomy during childbirth. In December of 2007, the National Institutes of Health issued a recommendation that episiotomies should only be performed when there are signs of fetal distress, meaning that the baby needs to be born quickly to avoid problems. If labor is proceeding normally, an episiotomy to cut vaginal tissues is unwarranted. If you have bowel incontinence, talk with your doctor about finding a specialist in bowel training. For many patients, the strength of the anal sphincter muscles can be improved through exercise. Surgery is available but only for severe cases. Read the lifestyle tips for living with urinary incontinence in chapter 9. They'll help you with your condition as well!

constipation worse. Bentyl (dicyclomine) has been used for as long as I can remember. A newer medication, Levsin (hyoscyamine) is also available.

Medications for Diarrhea

Imodium, a synthetic narcotic derivative, is available over the counter, but use it with caution. Because it is an opiate, it can be addictive and should be taken only as directed. (See "Diarrhea," below, for more information.)

Medications for Anxiety and Depression

Stress can cause colon spasms in people with IBS. The colon is densely packed with nerves that communicate constantly with the brain. These nerves control the normal contractions of the colon and can cause abdominal problems. Some of the older antidepressants such as Elavil and Norpramin can cause constipation, but if you are depressed and also have diarrhea, they may be just what you need.

Serotonin Blockers

As I explained, an excess of serotonin in the GI tract may be responsible for IBS symptoms. A medication now available specifically to treat IBS is alosetron hydrochloride (Lotronex). Lotronex has been reapproved with significant restrictions by the FDA for women with severe IBS who have not responded to conventional therapy and whose primary symptom is diarrhea. However, Lotronex should be used with great caution because it can have serious side effects such as severe constipation or decreased blood flow to the colon.

DIARRHEA

Diarrhea is a symptom, not a disease. Almost everybody has had one or more episodes of sudden, acute diarrhea often accompanied by vomiting. The cause is usually what we popularly refer to as "food poisoning" or "the twenty-four-hour flu" although the influenza virus doesn't cause this nuisance ailment. Your body is trying to get rid of whatever germ or toxin it is that has attacked your intestinal system. This type of gastroenteritis usually lasts one or two days and goes away on its own without special treatment. Prolonged diarrhea lasting more than two days may be a sign of a more serious problem, so you need to see a doctor. One possibility is dysentery, either amebic or bacillary, although these illnesses are typically found only in developing countries. You may also

Does the "Five-Second Rule" Work?

Maybe, maybe not. A team of researchers at Clemson University in South Carolina found that even if you pick up food that has been dropped on the floor within five seconds, it will have bacteria on it. However—no surprise here—it will have fewer bacteria than it would have if you had left it on the floor longer. So will following the five-second rule keep you from getting sick? Who knows? The study didn't involve having anyone eat any of the contaminated food. My call? I'd advise you to throw away any food that's been on the floor if only because that's good etiquette!

have one of the conditions we've already discussed in this chapter such as IBS and IBD.

SIGNS OF DIARRHEA

- loose, watery stools
- frequent stools
- dehydration symptoms including flushing and a dry mouth

CAUSES OF DIARRHEA

- Bacterial infections. Several types of bacteria consumed through contaminated food or water can cause diarrhea including campylobacter, salmonella, shigella, and strains of E. coli. The bacterium called Clostridium difficile or "C diff" most often affects older adults in hospitals and long-term-care facilities, especially those on antibiotics. Not only diarrhea but also a life-threatening inflammation of the colon can result.
- Parasitic infections. Parasites can enter the body through food or water and settle in the digestive system. Those that

cause diarrhea include giardia, Entamoeba histolytica, and cryptosporidium.

- Viral infections. Many viruses cause diarrhea including rotavirus, Norwalk virus, cytomegalovirus, herpes simplex virus, and viral hepatitis.
- Food intolerances. Some people are unable to digest food components such as artificial sweeteners, lactose, and gluten.
- Antibiotics. These can cause everything from mild diarrhea and temporary lactose intolerance to a dangerous toxic bowel inflammation called pseudomembranous colitis caused by the C. difficile toxin.
- Antacids containing magnesium
- Intestinal diseases. Inflammatory bowel disease, colitis, Crohn's disease, and celiac disease often lead to diarrhea. (See sidebar on IBS and IBD earlier in this chapter.)
- Irritable bowel syndrome (see the section on IBS earlier in this chapter)

Does Mayonnaise Cause Food Poisoning?

No, that's an old wives' tale. In fact a study published in the *Journal of Food Protection* showed that because mayonnaise is acidic, it actually helps keep bacteria from "spoiling" food. If you get sick from eating the second half of a tuna salad sandwich that you stashed in the glove compartment for several hours, the tuna is to blame. Be careful not to leave meat, fish, poultry, and eggs at room temperature for more than a short time. During barbecue season, keep food out of the sun and get it on the grill promptly. Another tip: Thaw frozen food in the refrigerator rather than on the counter, and then cook it right away.

Why Does the New Diet Drug "Alli" Cause Diarrhea?

Alli, the only FDA-approved over-the-counter diet drug, works by blocking digestion of fat. Any fat that you eat simply "goes right through you." If you cheat on the recommended low-fat diet, even a little bit, you'll end up with an embarrassing case of "the runs." Alli was advertised like crazy and thousands of people have tried it. However, a quick check of the Blogosphere turned up scores of posts from women complaining about "Alli diarrhea." One woman wrote, "Don't forget to take several changes of underwear with you wherever you go!" Ugh. That's a heavy price to pay for paring off a few pounds. Also, why tinker with the intricate healthy functioning of your gastrointestinal tract?

My advice is to establish healthy eating habits and get plenty exercise. If you need support, join a group such as Weight Watchers. A diet drug is not the answer even if it's been given the government's blessing! Furthermore, orlistat, another new drug, and Alli can block absorption of the fat-soluble vitamin D. With mounting evidence that most Americans don't have enough of this sunshine vitamin, this is another reason to skip the temptation to diet this way.

TREATMENT FOR ACUTE DIARRHEA
Diet

Until diarrhea goes away, usually within a day or two, avoid caffeine, all milk products including cheese and ice cream, and foods that are high in fiber, especially insoluble fiber, or "roughage." I recommend the soft, bland foods in the "BRAT" diet: **B**ananas, **R**ice, **A**pple juice, **T**oast. Drink only unsweetened juice and for now use white rice and white bread even though you're better off in general with the fiber and nutrients in brown rice and other whole grains. You can also eat boiled

What Is Traveler's Diarrhea?

If you travel abroad, in particular to developing countries with contaminated water supplies, you're at risk for traveler's diarrhea—also dubbed Montezuma's revenge and the "tourist trots." Follow my dos and don'ts to prevent an attack.

DO
- Drink bottled water, but only if you are the one to break the seal.
- Take antibiotics with you just in case. In fact your doctor may recommend that you take antibiotics before leaving to protect you from possible infection. I suggest traveling with a three-day supply of Cipro/500 mg to be taken twice daily at the first sign of GI distress or diarrhea. This treats E. coli, the most likely bacterial culprit, and other bacteria as well.

DON'T
- Drink tap water or use it to brush your teeth.
- Use ice made from tap water.
- Drink unpasteurized milk or dairy products.
- Eat raw fruits and vegetables unless they can be peeled and you peel them yourself.
- Eat raw or rare meat and fish.
- Eat meat or shellfish that isn't hot when served.
- Eat food from street vendors (I had the worst case of Montezuma's revenge ever from the most delicious frozen fruit bars ever in Mexico!)

skinless potatoes, plain crackers such as saltines, cooked carrots, and baked or poached chicken without the skin or fat.

Medications

If you have blood in your stool or possible antibiotic-related colitis, do not take the over-the-counter medication called Imodium (see "Medications for Diarrhea" on page 258). Imodium can cause a dangerous paralysis of your bowel.

If you have bacterial diarrhea, your doctor may prescribe antibiotics. I recommend three days of Cipro/500 mg, one twice daily. (See the sidebar on previous page.)

In many cases, you're best off not taking any medication to stop the diarrhea. As unpleasant as the condition is, it's your body's way of cleansing the GI tract of the "bugs." If you can stay home where you're close to your own bathroom, let the diarrhea run its course. Most people are too sick with diarrhea for a few days to go to work or school anyway.

Rehydration

As soon as you can keep fluids down, drink salty broths that will help hold water in your system. This will restore your electrolytes, including potassium. You can also buy over-the-counter rehydration products such as Pedialyte. These are marketed for children but adults can use them as well. If you are severely dehydrated to the point of feeling dizzy and faint, go to the emergency room. You may need to get fluids intravenously. Milk and dairy (lactose-containing products) should be the last thing you add back to your diet because many diarrheal illnesses cause a temporary lactose-intolerance that make bloating and diarrhea worse. Most yogurt is all right to eat since it contains the lactose-digesting bacteria acidophilus.

That wraps it up for bowel troubles. Now we'll move on to the urinary tract, another area "down there" that's prone to annoying and embarrassing problems. But take heart! As always, I'll teach you ways to deal with symptoms and I'll also let you know when you need to get professional help.

9

Internal Plumbing Down There

Urinary Troubles from Cause to Cure

IN THIS CHAPTER
- How Your Urinary Tract Is Supposed to Work
- How Colorful Is Your Water?
- Urinary Tract Infections
- Urinary Incontinence

According to the American Urological Association, approximately 40 percent of women have had "honeymoon cystitis," the searingly painful urinary tract infection that's most often triggered by intercourse. Add to that the estimated 30 percent of women who are dealing with an entirely different problem—long-term difficulty controlling urine—and the total number of women of all ages who've experienced one or both of these conditions is staggering. Cystitis is an infection that can lead to serous complications if left untreated, while the other condition, called incontinence, includes symptoms ranging from occasional embarrassing leaks to total loss of control that requires wearing a diaper. Together they constitute a huge health problem "down there." Yet, trust me, there are effective treatment options and strategies for both of these internal plumbing problems.

Needless to say, you're not going to feel particularly sexy if you end up with either or both of those all too common health issues. One of my patients, a thirty-five-year-old mother of two, put it this way: "I was at the point where I would get an infection practically every time my husband and I had sex. I got so I would find excuses whenever he came on to me."

Another woman, a doctor now in her fifties with three grown sons, had suffered in silence ever since childbirth had compromised her ability to hold her urine. "I'll never forget the time I made the mistake of drinking a super-sized soda right before we got in the car for a long drive to the beach," she said. "We ran into traffic on the expressway. When we finally got to an exit and pulled into a gas station, I realized it was too late. There was no time to ask for the bathroom key. I peed right there on the asphalt. Talk about being mortified!" Her urinary problems extended to the bedroom in that she felt she needed to shower before lovemaking in case any dribbles had left an odor. She also always worried that sex might prompt a leak. That concern pulled focus from her pleasure.

Full disclosure: I was the second woman. For years, I was as guilty as the next woman of not talking about my problem and not looking for solutions even though as a doctor I was successfully treating other women with this problem. That all changed when I shared my story with other women. The simple act of letting my friends in on my urinary problem went a long way toward making me feel better about it. In fact, many of my friends admitted that they also had this problem. There's nothing like a good laugh with a girlfriend to put a situation such as this one in perspective! I encourage you, too, to be more open about any urinary problems and also to tell your primary care physician or your gynecologist about the issue in order to get help. (See chapter 3 for advice about how to talk with your physician as well as information on how to keep a health journal and make lists of symptoms and questions to prepare for office visits.) The good news is that there are simple and affordable ways to deal with most urinary tract problems and that there are effective treatments for the more serious conditions. I'm going to share this information with you so that you can reclaim your love life—and for that matter, enjoy your whole life more! The journey begins with learning exactly how urination works.

HOW YOUR URINARY TRACT
IS SUPPOSED TO WORK

Our kidneys remove waste and excess water from the bloodstream in the form of urine, which passes from the kidneys to the bladder through long, thin tubes called ureters, then from the bladder out of the body through a much shorter tube called the urethra. We make urine constantly, and lots of it—about four or five cups in twenty-four hours. It stays in our own personal storage bag (the bladder) thanks to three sets of muscles: 1) sphincter muscles that pinch off the top of the urethra to keep urine from leaving the bladder; 2) pelvic floor muscles that pinch off the bottom of the urethra to keep urine from leaking out of the body; and 3) muscles in the bladder wall.

The bladder, bladder neck, and urethra are held in place by an elaborate system of muscles called the pelvic sling or pelvic floor; nerves that direct the muscles to contract and relax; and ligaments, which hold up the bladder by attaching to bones and other structures. (See the drawing of the "pelvic sling" in chapter 1.)

Here's how everything is supposed to work: When your bladder begins to fill up, it sends messages to the brain that you "gotta go." The brain is remarkably good at detecting when you are in a safe place to go and holds off sending the "okay to empty" command until then. That's why most of us don't wet the bed at night despite having a full bladder. Once you're on the toilet and you get the go-ahead from your brain, your sphincter and pelvic floor muscles—the "pinch-tight" muscles—relax so that the entire length of your urethra is open. Then the muscles in your bladder wall contract, forcing the urine down the urethra and out of your body. After the urine drains, the pinch-tight muscles close so that the bladder bag can fill up again.

If everything is nice and tight and in proper position, we maintain control over when and how we urinate. When we cough, sneeze, or laugh, the urethra is pulled up against the supports and stays tightly closed. However, like most body functions, urination is not always perfect.

HOW COLORFUL IS YOUR WATER?

The color of your urine can tell a lot about your diet or general state of health. Always talk with your doctor if your urine changes color dramatically. Although most of the time a change in color can be traced to food or pharmaceutical dyes, it is sometimes an early sign of a health problem.

- Clear to pale yellow. This is the normal color urine in a person who is healthy and well hydrated.
- Dark yellow to orange. Darker urine is a sign of dehydration. Without enough water to dilute urine, the yellow color is intensified. Dehydration can be dangerous. Make sure you drink enough fluids. If you have a medical condition such as diarrhea or food poisoning, call your doctor. You may need intravenous fluids. Darker urine can also be caused by the supplements vitamin B2 and beta carotene, but the spectrum in these cases is from orange to a bright, almost fluorescent yellow. In addition, eating large amounts of rhubarb may turn urine orange. Pyridium, an oral medication for symptomatic relief of urinary tract infections, can also turn your urine orange and can even stain panties if you leak urine. None of these causes are harmful.
- Red or pink. Eating lots of beets can turn urine slightly red. However, redness is often a sign of having blood in the urine. This could indicate a simple urinary tract infection or it may be a sign of a serious kidney problem. Anyone with red or pink urine should contact a doctor.

- Blue or green. Asparagus can lend a light green tint and a pungent odor to urine. People who are genetically programmed to have high levels of blood calcium (hypercalcemia) also have blue-green urine.
- Brown. Bile from the liver can turn urine brown, anywhere from light weak-tea brown to a dark chestnut brown. Because brownish urine can be an indicator of muscle breakdown, hepatitis, a bile blockage from a stone, or liver disease, you should go to your primary care physician for an examination as well as blood work and a urinalysis. Depending on the results, you may get a referral to a specialist. In rare cases, when statin medications for cholesterol cause muscle breakdown, your urine turns cola-colored. This signals a potential medical emergency. You should stop the medication immediately and be treated in the hospital with plenty of fluids.

URINARY TRACT INFECTIONS

Escherichia coli (E. coli) bacteria are almost always the culprits when it comes to urinary tract infections (UTI). Everyone has E. coli in the colon and the bacteria don't do any harm there. However, they *can* cause an infection if they manage to get into your urinary tract. I'll spell out for you the ways that can happen, but first I want to explain what we mean by UTI.

As you learned in chapter 1, the urethra and bladder are called the lower urinary tract while the ureters and kidneys are called the upper urinary tract. An infection of the lower tract is called "cystitis." The word comes from "cyst," which means "empty vessel" and refers to the bladder, and "itis," which is a medical suffix meaning "inflammation of." An inflammation is the body's response to infection or injury. The symptoms are swelling, warmth, redness, and pain.

An infection of the upper urinary tract is called "pyelonephritis." Also, a chronic condition characterized by pelvic pain, urinary urgency, and fatigue is called "interstitial cystitis." Neither one of these conditions is as common as lower urinary tract cystitis. That may be why doctors and patients alike tend to use the terms UTI and cystitis interchangeably. This is true even if a woman has a lower urinary tract inflammation that was caused by a minor injury or an irritant but she hasn't developed an infection. Technically, however, the terms "acute bacterial cystitis" and "pyelonephritis" fall under the umbrella term of UTI and the terms "noninfectious cystitis" and "chronic interstitial cystitis" refer to the urinary tract conditions that don't involve infections.

Of course, whatever you call your condition, it hurts and it's a surefire libido buster. Here's what you need to know about the symptoms, causes, treatment, and prevention so you can get well and stay that way.

HOW TO TELL IF YOU HAVE CYSTITIS
Symptoms of Cystitis

- frequent, urgent need to urinate
- burning pain when you start and stop urinating
- pressure or discomfort just above your pelvic bone
- backache
- urine that is cloudy, bloody, or foul-smelling

Diagnostic Tests
Over-the-Counter Urine Test Strips
You can buy these strips at any drugstore without a prescription. If you follow the instructions and the results show nitrates in your urine, that is a sign of the presence of bacteria. If your test results also show white blood cells in your urine, you almost certainly have an infection that needs to be treated.

Test Name	Results	Units	Reference Range	Site
336 URINALYSIS				
SPECIFIC GRAVITY	1.026		1.005- 1.035	
COLOR	YELLOW		YELLOW	
APPEARANCE	CLEAR		CLEAR	
PH	6.5		4.5- 8.0	
GLUCOSE,QL	NEGATIVE		NEGATIVE	
PROTEIN,TOTAL,QL	NEGATIVE		NEGATIVE	
KETONES	NEGATIVE		NEGATIVE	
HEMOGLOBIN,QL	NEGATIVE		NEGATIVE	
LEUKOCYTE ESTERASE	NEGATIVE		NEGATIVE	
BILIRUBIN	NEGATIVE		NEGATIVE	
NITRITE	NEGATIVE		NEGATIVE	
WBC	0-5	PER HPF	0- 5	
RBC	0-3	PER HPF	0- 3	
EPITHELIAL CELLS	FEW SQUAMOUS EPITHELIAL CELLS		FEW/MOD. SQUAMOUS	
CRYSTALS	AMORPHOUS URATE CRYSTALS OBSERVED			

Urinalysis results

Urinalysis

An analysis performed in your doctor's office or a lab with a dipstick is done for the same reason as the home test. Your doctor can also look at your urine under the microscope or send the sample to a laboratory to confirm the presence of bacteria, white blood cells, and red blood cells and to look for other signs of kidney disease.

Urine Culture

A urine culture done in a lab confirms the diagnosis of cystitis by verifying that a significant amount of bacteria is present in your urine. Eighty to 90 percent of the time, the bacteria are E. coli. However, on occasion other bacteria from the colon, such as enterococcus, proteus, or pseudomonas, may be causing the infection. The test results will help determine which antibiotics will work for you. Your urine is put in a petri dish along with a nutrient broth. If bacteria are present, they will grow. The lab technician will count the number of colonies of bacteria and report this information to your doctor. If your urine contains

What Is the Difference between External and Internal Dysuria?

Dysuria is the medical term for pain with urination. Internal dysuria refers to pain you experience when your urine is on the way out and your urethra is inflamed from cystitis (see chapter 7). External dysuria is the stinging sensation you feel when urine touches your vulvar skin. You may have fissures (cracks in the skin) or possibly blisters from an infection such as HSV-2 or yeast vulvovaginitis (see chapter 2).

multiple types of bacteria in small amounts, then the sample may have been contaminated and will need to be repeated.

CAUSES OF CYSTITIS

With noninfectious cystitis, the cause is an irritation of your urethra that leads to an inflammation. With acute bacterial cystitis, E. coli from your colon are transferred from your anus to your nearby urethra by any number of means, most often a free ride on your partner's penis. Then the E. coli happily travel up your urethra and try to set up shop in your normally sterile bladder. If they succeed, you get an infection. The infection subsequently causes an inflammation.

The E. coli don't always succeed, though. The bladder is a pretty unfriendly environment for bacteria. Urine is very acidic and that keeps bacteria from growing. Most of the time when bacteria enter the bladder, they don't set up housekeeping and are flushed out during urination. However, this natural infection protection depends on the balanced functioning of the whole urinary tract. The balance can be upset by changes in diet, immune problems, stress, poorly controlled diabetes, menopause, and incomplete emptying of the bladder that leads to stagnating residual urine. When the balance is out of whack, bacteria are able to stay in the bladder and reproduce. (They do so very quickly. E. coli divide and multiply every twenty minutes.) Eventually the bacteria could travel up the ureter and into the kidney, but lower urinary tract cystitis is so painful so soon that women usually get treatment long before the E. coli have a chance to cause an upper urinary tract infection.

Here are the typical triggers of cystitis:

Sex

Cystitis is not classified as a sexually transmitted disease (STD), but vigorous sex and frequent sex can have a double whammy effect. First, you can get an inflammation as a result of minor trauma when the penis rubs your urethra. You can also get an infection and subsequent inflammation if E. coli are transferred from your vulvar skin to your urethra and bladder. The term "honeymoon cystitis" is actually a misnomer because the problem can happen whenever you and your partner get a little extra frisky between the sheets. Then too, any sexual activity can cause cystitis, especially if a health problem such as a weakened immune system or diabetes leaves you prone to contracting an infection.

Not Changing Your Sanitary Pad or Panty Liner Often Enough

Prolonged contact with a moist environment encourages bacteria to grow and to pass from the rectal area to the urethra. Using maxi pads when your flow is especially heavy is fine, but change the pads often. Never use maxi pads simply to prolong the time between changes when your flow is light. Panty liners can also bring on cystitis if you leave them on twenty-four/seven. Even a dry panty liner can be enough of an irritant to cause urinary problems.

How to Give "Good" Urine

Urine cultures are often unreliable in women because the urine can easily be contaminated by the normal bacteria of the vagina or skin surrounding the urethra. That's why urine tests require that you give a "midstream clean catch" specimen. Here's what you do:

1. Open the packet containing an antibacterial wipe. Do not let the wipe touch any bathroom surface. If you accidentally drop it, ask for another one.

2. Wipe the area of your vulva and urethra, including the surrounding skin, with the antibacterial wipe. Wipe from front to back. Once you wipe, do not touch your skin with your fingers.

3. Open the sealed packet containing the sterile cup. Do not let the inside of the cup touch any surface in the bathroom, and do not touch the lip of the cup with your fingers. There will also be a cap for the cup. Do not let the cap touch any bathroom surface either.

4. Urinate into the toilet for about three seconds, then place the cup into the urine stream and collect a sample that fills the cup half to three-quarters full. If you haven't finished urinating, allow the remainder to fall into the toilet. This step is trickier than it sounds. Don't be surprised if you feel like a contortionist with Cirque du Soleil, or if you end up with urine dribbling down your hand. (It is also possible that you'll freeze up for a bit. Usually I can pee on command, yet when I put a cup under me suddenly my brain won't let it happen!)

5. Cap the cup, being careful not to touch the lip of the cup with your fingers.

6. Write your name on the cup and leave it where instructed.

Feminine Hygiene Products and Bubble Baths

Douches, sprays, and bubble baths have chemicals that can irritate your urethra.

Diaphragms and Spermicidal Gels

These can both irritate your urethra.

A Genetic Condition

A study done by researchers at the Northwestern University Medical School in Chicago has shown that women with recurrent cystitis may have receptors in the bladder to which E. coli adhere easily, making bladder infection more common.

Menopause

As a result of reduced estrogen after menopause, vaginal bacteria change from friendly lactobacillus to bacteria types similar to the E. coli in your colon. Menopause also causes the urethra and the clitoris to atrophy, or shrink. Before menopause the urethra's cushion of estrogen-rich tissue acts like a door, closing the opening of the urethra. After menopause it's thinner and less effective at keeping the urethra closed making post-menopausal women especially prone to cystitis.

Diabetes

Poorly controlled diabetes (in which the blood sugar is too high) interferes with immune function and leads to susceptibility to all kinds of infections, including cystitis.

Wiping from Back to Front

If you wipe from back to front, you'll spread stool with E. coli and other bacteria in it to the urethra.

Asymptomatic Bacteriuria and Pregnant Women

Some people have bacteria in their urine with no symptoms. This is called asymptomatic bacteriuria, or asymptomatic UTI. The condition is not usually a cause for concern and most often requires no treatment. However, in pregnant women it can lead to serious kidney infections and may cause premature birth. That's one of the reasons obstetricians ask pregnant women for a urine sample at nearly every office visit.

TREATING CYSTITIS

A number of antibiotics are effective in curing cystitis. A 2002 report in the *Archives of Internal Medicine* offered guidelines to doctors for deciding whether to prescribe antibiotics. If you have any two of the following three criteria, you are a candidate for antibiotics even without going for an office visit or having a urine culture: 1) painful or difficult urination, 2) urinalysis results that show white blood cells in your urine, 3) urinalysis results that show nitrates in your urine. In other words, if you have painful or difficult urination and your home urine strip test (described on page 270) meets even one more of the three criteria, your doctor can call in a prescription to your pharmacy. Otherwise, you'll need to go to your doctor's office for a urinalysis and a urine culture.

If antibiotics are prescribed, take them. You may be tempted to try to flush the infection out of your system by drinking lots of cranberry juice and other fluids, but with cystitis, taking antibiotics reduces the likelihood of future infections.

You won't have to take antibiotics for very long in order to get rid of the infection. I used to prescribe a single dose of antibiotics. That did make the symptoms go away, but often the infection wasn't totally eliminated and it flared up again. A three-day regimen is usually all that is needed if the right antibiotic is chosen, for example Bactrim or Cipro. (I don't recommend Cipro. See the sidebar on page 280.) However, my choice has long been a five- to seven-day regimen with Macrodantin. A 2008 review of treatment for cystitis corroborated my belief that Macrodantin is the best first bet. It works and it won't promote yeast infections. Tetracyclines such as doxycycline or minocycline were commonly used in the past as seven-day regimens, but 80 percent of women who take them will develop a yeast infection so it's best to avoid them.

The seven-day regimen is best for women with diabetes but for most women the three-day regimen carries less risk of side effects such as headaches, nausea, and a vaginal yeast infection that could result if the antibiotics knock out the healthy bacteria in the vagina. Some women with frequent yeast infections will automatically start using yeast creams to avoid a yeast infection whenever they are prescribed antibiotics for any reason, and this works.

If you still have painful and urgent urination after you have finished your antibiotic therapy, make an appointment for a urinalysis and urine culture. You may need a different antibiotic than the one you were taking and you may need to take it for as long as two weeks. While you're waiting for your antibiotic to kick in, your doctor may prescribe a medication called Pyridium (phenazopyridine) that eases the pain you feel when you urinate and also lessens your urgency and frequency. (Remember, I mentioned before that this drug changes the color of your urine). This drug is not an antibiotic and it does not cure infections. The usual dose is one 200-milligram tablet two or three times daily after meals. I have occasionally given my patients prescriptions for this medication to take along when they're traveling, in case they need immediate relief from cystitis and can't get antibiotics right away. However, the sooner

Antibiotics for Cystitis

Although research into antibiotics is continually evolving, these are my favorite treatments for cystitis.

- **Bactrim** (trimethoprim-sulfamethoxazole). Bactrim is a popular and highly effective medication for cystitis. However, bacteria are developing a resistance to this drug so if you've taken it recently, it may no longer work and you'll need to take a different antibiotic. Also, you can't take this drug if you're allergic to sulfa, since that's an ingredient in this combination drug. (The first sign of an allergic reaction is a bright red rash. If you develop a rash, call your doctor.)
- **Amoxicillin and Keflex** (cephalexin). These work, but only if you have certain strains of E. coli and other colon bacteria. They also upset your vaginal balance of bacteria, leading to one in four women getting yeast vaginitis. If you are allergic to penicillin, you can't take either one of these.
- **Augmentin** (amoxicillin-clavulanate). This is usually effective, but it's expensive and is also to be avoided if you are allergic to penicillin.
- **Macrodantin** (nitrofurantoin). This antibiotic has been around for as long as I can remember and remains highly effective against E. coli and won't disturb your vaginal flora, so it doesn't pose any increased risk of yeast infections. A recent study in the Archives of Internal Medicine found that five days of nitrofurantoin is as good as three days of Bactrim, so this is often my first choice if patients are allergic to sulfa (a component of Bactrim) or have been treated with Bactrim recently.

you start taking antibiotics the better. Please remember that. Don't be fooled into thinking you're fine just because Pyridium is masking your symptoms. The longer you wait to take antibiotics, the longer you'll have to take antibiotics to get rid of the infection. You are also putting yourself at risk for a serious kidney infection.

TREATING RECURRENT CYSTITIS

If your cystitis comes back time after time, the first question you and your doctor should ask is whether this is a relapse or a reinfection. Relapse means the infection never went away completely even though your symptoms subsided for a while. It may also mean that the antibiotic you were taking no longer works for you. You will need to start taking an antibiotic again, perhaps a different one from the one you took the first time. Also, you will almost certainly need to take the antibiotic for seven days or even longer.

If several months have elapsed since your first bout of cystitis, you have been reinfected with another strain of E. coli or other bacteria. In other words, your original infection was cured but you got another one. Some women have up to seven infections per year. Sometimes women go through periods in their lives when they have infections frequently, but then the infections gradually stop occurring.

If you have more than three episodes of cystitis a year, I recommend that you try these simple preventive measures:

- Immediately after having sex, get up to urinate in order to flush out any bacteria.
- If you are using a diaphragm and spermicidal jelly, consider other forms of birth control because these can irritate the urethra. (Of course, if this is the only reasonable contraceptive option for you, please continue using it.)
- If you often take painkillers that contain acetaminophen, such as Tylenol, cut back since they may be making you susceptible to cystitis.

Do You Recommend Cipro?

I am not recommending as a first choice the commonly prescribed and expensive Cipro (100 mg twice daily) and Floxacin (200 mg twice daily) antibiotics although they are highly effective. The more you take these antibiotics, called fluoroquinolones, the more likely you are to build up immunity to their effectiveness. Since these drugs are also useful for life-threatening infections (remember the anthrax scare?) I prefer to save them for when you're fighting something serious.

- Drink lots of cranberry juice. Studies show it can reduce the number of infections. Although cranberry juice acidifies urine, which could help reduce bacteria growth, current thinking is that cranberry juice contains a chemical that prevents bacteria from attaching to the cells that line the urethra and bladder. Keep in mind that a "cranberry juice cocktail" contains sugars and other juices that do nothing to combat cystitis. You need to find pure cranberry juice in order to get the full benefit of this remedy. Also, you may be tempted to try the popular chewable cranberry tablets such as CranActin, but be warned that they are expensive and that scientists don't know if they work as well as cranberry juice.
- If your infections typically happen as a result of having sex, with symptoms occurring in a matter of hours or even less after intercourse, ask your doctor if she will prescribe a low dose of an antibiotic as a preventive measure. I prescribe a half a tablet of Bactrim for my patients who are good candidates for this drug. At a dose this low, you lower the risk of having bacteria resistant to Bactrim. I advise my patients to take it right before or after having sex, up to three times per week. This is almost always

effective and it's definitely safe if you are not allergic to sulfa-containing drugs such as Bactrim. I recommend continuing this regimen for six months and then stopping the medication. If the infections recur, you can go back on the medication.

- If you have fewer than three infections a year, ask your doctor if she will give you a prescription to keep on hand so that you can start a short course of antibiotics such as Bactrim or Macrodantin at the first sign of an infection without a visit to the doctor or a urine culture. Keep a written record of each time you have

Why Does Cystitis Keep Coming Back after Menopause?

Decreased estrogen after menopause can cause your vulvar tissue to thin or "shrink" and have a tendency to become easily inflamed. This condition is called atrophic vaginitis and it can contribute to frequent bouts of cystitis. Ask your doctor about prescribing a topical estrogen cream if that is an option for you (see chapter 7). Although a number of studies have shown that using estrogen does not significantly reduce the chance of getting cystitis, I am not convinced. I have found that using a small dose of vaginal estrogen cream or even using a minute amount of the cream around the urethra opening can make a big difference for me and for many of my patients. If only you could see the changes that I see! When treated with estrogen, a woman who has severe atrophic vaginitis—with thin, pale tissue with the urethra somewhat opened—has her urethra become moist, pink, thickened, and no longer "open." That's an amazing difference! If your doctor will give you a prescription, the cream is worth a try. You can always stop using the cream if it doesn't work for you.

Diagnostic Tests for the Urinary Tract

Kidney ultrasound: A kidney and pelvic ultrasound is a great first bet. It is noninvasive, easy, painless, requires no preparation, and can reveal a lot of potential problems. The ultrasound uses sound waves to visualize the pelvic organs and kidneys so the doctor can look for the presence of cysts, kidney size, and blockage from scar tissue from previous infections. An ultrasound is not as good for identifying kidney stones, however.

Intravenous pyelogram (IVP): An IVP is valuable for showing stones or other blockages in ureters or anywhere else along the kidney system. IVP involves injecting dye into the veins and then taking a series of X-rays that follow the progress of the dye through the kidneys and out the body. These pictures show minute detail not only of your kidney size but how your kidneys function. The kidney and ureters and bladder "light up," so to speak, so your doctor gets more detailed pictures than with an ultrasound. Before ultrasound became so widespread, IVP was the most frequent test for figuring out why cystitis keeps recurring. *NOTE:* The dye contains iodine and some people are allergic to it. There's no way to test for an allergic reaction before the first time you have the dye injected into your veins. A medical team will be at the ready with systemic antihistamine and adrenaline to administer at the first sign that you are having a reaction. This will ensure that you don't go into shock. Of course, once you know you're allergic to iodine, tell your doctor not to give you this test and add this allergy to the list on the emergency health information card you keep in your wallet (see chapter 3).

> **Cystoscopy:** This is a test that allows a urologist to look inside the bladder by passing a tiny light on a long, flexible cord into the urethra. As you might imagine, local anesthesia is required. A cystoscopy can pick up things the other tests might miss, such as large bladder stones, hidden sacks called diverticula that are full of bacteria or infection, and even cancer (although cancer is quite unlikely to be the cause of cystitis).

symptoms and the name and dose of the antibiotic along with the results of your treatment. Research has shown that this approach is safe and effective so your doctor should be happy to comply with your request.

If your infections keep recurring in spite of preventive measures and continued treatment, you will need a more intensive investigation to find out why this is happening. Tests will be done to look for problems that might make you more likely to have recurrent infections. You may already have progressive asymptomatic ("silent") kidney disease that needs to be treated.

For example, chronic kidney or bladder stones can be a source of ongoing infection. If you have recurrent stones, you may get a referral to see a urologist to have them removed. Another more conservative option is to get a referral to see a kidney specialist, called a nephrologist, who can discuss medication treatment that could decrease your chance of developing future stones.

Polycystic kidney disease, a genetic disorder in which multiple cysts grow on the kidneys, is often linked to frequent urinary tract infections and the disease can eventually cause kidney failure. However, there are treatment options that can be tried long before that happens. You will be referred to a nephrologist.

Other possible causes of recurrent cystitis include undiagnosed diabetes, structural blockage from scarring from previous infections, endometriosis, Crohn's disease, and congenital abnormalities in the shape and size of your kidneys or ureters.

CAUSES OF PYELONEPHRITIS

Bacterial Cystitis That Spreads to the Upper Urinary Tract

If you have symptoms of cystitis—such as urgent, painful urination—and you delay getting medical attention, you put yourself at risk for giving the E. coli time to travel up to your kidneys. Heed your body's warning signs and contact a doctor fast.

Anatomical Abnormalities

You may have been born with small or misshapen kidneys or short ureters. These anomalies can allow bacteria to get to your kidneys more quickly than normal so that you end up with a kidney infection even before you get help for cystitis. Children can develop a temporary reflux or backwash of urine from the bladder up the ureters that leads to frequent infections and potentially to kidney scarring if not treated promptly with antibiotics. Fortunately this ureteral reflux usually disappears when children grow. Ureteral reflux is the most common cause of cystitis in children.

HOW TO TELL IF YOU HAVE PYELONEPHRITIS

Some women who have a lower urinary tract infection also have an asymptomatic or "silent" infection of the kidney. Doctors don't typically look for it since the antibiotics prescribed for cystitis usually knock out the kidney infection as well. However, if the antibiotics don't cure the pyelonephritis, symptoms of the lingering infection typically occur suddenly (see below). This is a serious condition and you should call your doctor immediately. You will almost certainly need to be hospitalized in order to be given antibiotics and fluids intravenously.

Symptoms of Pyelonephritis

- fever
- lower-back or kidney-area pain
- chills
- shaking
- nausea
- vomiting
- inability to urinate

INTERSTITIAL CYSTITIS

A chapter on bladder problems in women wouldn't be complete without at least a mention of the debilitating but fortunately not too common condition called interstitial cystitis (IC) or painful bladder syndrome. This condition was not even recognized when I was in school but it is finally getting attention. However, it remains difficult to treat and incredibly frustrating for women who have it. IC is characterized by pelvic pain, urinary urgency, urinary frequency, nocturia (frequent need to urinate during the night), painful intercourse, and pain or discomfort while sitting for a long time in a car or at a desk.

The cause of IC is unknown. Urine cultures are typically negative for infection. A number of treatment options have been tried without much success. Most recently, however, a drug called pentosan polysulfate placed directly in the bladder has been shown to be effective in easing the symptoms. A study by C. Lowell Parsons, M.D., a leading expert on IC, reported that 90 percent of the patients had reduced symptoms. If you are an IC sufferer, I hope you'll not only find relief from your symptoms but also a doctor who takes your symptoms seriously and is willing to work with you until you find a treatment that works for you!

Actually, that's my wish for all of you who have been struggling with any type of urinary tract infection or inflammation or any condition that seems to get too little attention or is not taken seriously. Now let's move on to the other urinary tract issue that plagues so many women. . . .

URINARY INCONTINENCE

Our ability to control urination is affected by everything that makes us women—menstruation, pregnancy, childbirth, and menopause. There are two types: stress incontinence and urge incontinence. The word "stress" doesn't refer to emotional stress. It means pressure on your bladder, such as when you laugh or cough or simply wait too long to urinate. You are "stressing" your bladder and urethra. The source of this problem is damage or weakening of the muscles of your pelvic floor. Although urinary tract infections and inflammations are marked by women complaining to their doctors of annoying and severe symptoms, incontinence is a condition that women tend to underreport or don't discuss at all.

Urge incontinence is also called irritable bladder syndrome, overactive bladder, and spastic bladder. When you have this condition, your bladder empties despite your best efforts to control it, even if it's not particularly full and you haven't waited very long between trips to the bathroom. The humorous direct-to-consumer television ads for urinary incontinence medications are aimed at women with urge incontinence. In the commercials women twist and shimmy around, desperate to get to the bathroom, all to the catchy jingle, "gotta go, gotta go, gotta go."

However, as any woman who has either variation of incontinence can tell you, the condition is no laughing matter. Who wants to publicize this very personal problem by standing in the checkout line at the drugstore holding a package of adult diapers? For this reason, a lot of women use menstrual pads to catch urine accidents, even though the pads are not as effective as diapers.

I know how much you want to conquer incontinence and do away with the need for any kind of protection. I can't promise you a 100 percent cure, but I can definitely help you gain a great deal more control. Let's start by having a look at the origins of incontinence.

CAUSES OF STRESS INCONTINENCE

Menstruation

A study done in 2002 by researchers at the Department of Epidemiology and Social Medicine in Aarhus, Denmark, showed that a significant number of women have episodes of stress incontinence between days eleven and fifteen of their menstrual cycles. They attribute this to ovulation when there is a lot of uterine tissue thickening your uterus and putting pressure on your bladder.

Pregnancy

The increasing weight of your uterus puts extra strain on your pelvic floor muscles and your bladder and also simply takes up space. Especially during your third trimester, you will probably leak a little when you laugh or cough. Also, your bladder doesn't have as much room to fill up, so you may feel the need to urinate fairly often and fairly urgently. Any woman who's been pregnant knows this. That's why if there's ever a long line for the ladies' room, we automatically let a pregnant woman cut to the front of the line!

Childbirth

Particularly if you have a long labor, you may end up with damage to the muscles and connective tissue of your pelvic floor. Other factors contributing to postpartum incontinence include the use of forceps and delivering a baby who weighs over eight pounds.

Menopause

A 2008 *New England Journal of Medicine* article on stress urinary incontinence by Rebecca G. Rogers, M.D., of the University of New Mexico Health Services Center reported that 25 percent of perimenopausal women and 40 percent of postmenopausal women report leakage of urine. Many of the women said they leak during sex. However, only half of these women talk to their doctors about the problem. If you're among that number, speak up! The causes of menopausal incontinence are lowered estrogen levels and aging pelvic muscles that are losing strength.

Fibroids

These are noncancerous growths of the uterus. (See chapter 7.)

Obesity

Belly fat puts pressure on your bladder.

Chronic Cough

Smoking, asthma, bronchitis, and blood pressure medications called ACE-inhibitors can all result in a frequent and persistent cough that puts pressure on your pelvic floor muscles.

Chronic Constipation

Straining to have a bowel movement can weaken the muscles of your pelvic floor.

Occupations or Recreational Activities That Cause Pressure on Your Bladder

Examples include waitressing (because you're on your feet for long periods), weight lifting at the gym, and aerobics.

Immobility

If you are bedridden or confined to a wheelchair, the muscles of your pelvic floor atrophy from lack of use.

Antihistamines and Antidepressants

Medications such as Benadryl, Elavil, and Tofranil have an "anticholinergic" effect, meaning that they inhibit contractions of certain muscle groups such as the bladder and colon. This can make it hard for you to fully empty your bladder (or colon for that matter). When there's a little extra urine left, it can leak out later. These drugs also blunt the "gotta go" signal, resulting in a very full bladder that's prone to leaking. These problems are temporary and will end when you go off the medication. (These drugs can also be a big problem in men with enlarged prostates, making urinating very difficult if they can go at all.)

Diuretics

Prescription and over-the-counter medications as well as caffeinated drinks and alcohol can lead to frequency and urgency. However, diuretics are often the best choice to treat high blood pressure as well as to prevent calcium-loaded kidney stones, so don't avoid them. I take them myself. You'll get used to a full bladder and the need to go frequently. Just do as I do and size up the location of the bathroom everywhere you go. Also, skipping a dose is safe if you know you'll be unable to get to a bathroom for several hours. I skip a dose when I have to tape long television segments or give speeches.

Brain Injuries

Stroke, multiple sclerosis, diabetes and Parkinson's disease can cause incontinence, primarily because of nerve rather than muscle damage.

Radiation for Cervical Cancer
This can cause injury to the bladder.

HOW TO TELL IF YOU HAVE STRESS INCONTINENCE
There's no need to have any diagnostic tests. You can be sure you have stress incontinence if you leak urine or have a full-on accident when you do any of the following:

- laugh
- cough
- sneeze
- jump
- have sex
- wait too long to find a bathroom

TREATING STRESS INCONTINENCE
Pelvic Floor Exercises
These exercises have long been known to be the single most effective treatment for minimizing stress incontinence. They are often referred to as Kegels, after Dr. Arnold Kegel, the gynecologist who created them in 1948. A review of clinical trials of pelvic floor exercises published in the October 2000 issue of *Obstetrics and Gynecology* showed that 61 percent of women who performed Kegels reported being "cured or almost cured." Just as with any other muscles, the mantra for pelvic floor muscles is "use it or lose it."

Your doctor can teach you how to find the muscles you need to exercise. She'll insert a gloved finger in your vagina and have you squeeze it. However, you can learn to find the correct muscles by yourself. While you're urinating, imagine that somebody startles you by opening the bathroom door. Your instinct will be to squeeze and stop the flow. If you are able to do that, you have contracted exactly the right muscles.

Just as you would if you were exercising your thigh muscles or your biceps, you need to do multiple repetitions to gain strength in your pelvic floor muscles. I recommend squeezing and holding for five seconds, then releasing and repeating for a total of ten repetitions. Do this three to five times a week. You will notice improvement in six to eight weeks. After three to six months you will probably be cured or almost cured. Also, after you've mastered the Kegel squeeze, you can do a strong contraction when you feel a cough or a sneeze coming on and you'll stand a good chance of preventing a leak. Kegels help your sex life, too, because you'll be able to squeeze voluntarily and thus heighten pleasure for both of you. However, to stay in shape, you'll need to continue doing the exercises on a regular basis.

Vaginal Weight Training

A vaginal cone is a weight about the size of a tampon that fits into your vagina. The cones come in sets of three to five graduated weights ranging from twenty to seventy grams. You start by inserting the lightest one and holding it there for fifteen minutes twice a day. After four to six weeks, you move up to the next heaviest weight and continue until you're able to use the heaviest weight. However, no studies have shown that using weights is any more effective than simply doing Kegels, and in fact Kegels are often shown to be more effective than using weights.

Diet

Pay attention to which foods and beverages tend to make you more prone to episodes of stress incontinence. Keeping a diet journal is one way to do this. Just about everyone with stress incontinence will end up with a list of trigger items that includes caffeine, spicy foods, acidic citrus fruits and juices, alcohol, and chocolate. However, you may find that other foods or beverages tend to irritate your bladder as well. Each of us reacts a little differently, which is why you are the best judge of what to avoid. On the other hand, you might want to consult a dietician or nutritionist who can keep you motivated.

You need enough water every day to make up for the losses in your urine and sweat, so don't be tempted to cut back there. Dehydration will concentrate your urine, which in turn will irritate your bladder. The trick is to time your fluid intake. Drink your glasses of water when you know you'll be able to get to a bathroom within a hour or so rather than right before a long drive or an evening at the theater where the line to the ladies' room is sure to be long. It goes without saying that you won't want to drink a lot of water right before going to bed.

Weight Loss

According to a clinical trial done at the University of Arkansas for Medical Sciences (UAMS) and published in the January 29, 2009 issue of the *New England Journal of Medicine*, losing weight helps women reduce the incidence of urinary incontinence. Of course losing weight is easier said than done. If you've tried time and again to pare off pounds without success, consider getting support from groups such as Weight Watchers or Overeaters Anonymous.

Biofeedback

Biofeedback is done via low frequency electrical stimulation of the pelvic floor with a vaginal or rectal probe. This method can help you if you're having trouble isolating your pelvic muscles in order to do pelvic floor exercises.

Surgery

There is a growing specialty in gynecologic urology that was spearheaded years ago by forward-thinking physicians. Among them was my late father-in-law, Dr. Arnold Fenton, who held the first chair in OB-GYN at North Shore University Hospital on Long Island. During his funeral in 2007, I learned that he was credited with seeing the importance of urology training for gynecologists many years ago and started one of the first GYN-Urology programs in the country. He had such a wonderful sensitivity and understanding of the needs of women in so many aspects of their health. These days gynecologic urologists are a great resource for women. Twenty years ago I wouldn't have recommended that you see a surgeon for stress incontinence because back then your only option would have been a urologist whose knowledge and practice was almost always limited to men. My sister Eileen underwent surgery for incontinence when she was in her thirties and ended up with several postoperative problems including intestinal blockage and difficulty moving her bowels. She also experienced very little improvement in her urine symptoms.

Today, however, I would encourage you to have a consultation with a gynecologic urologist. Surgical cases have doubled in the past decade as baby-boomer women have pushed doctors to find new ways to treat incontinence. There are more than 250 types of surgical techniques for incontinence. They vary from collagen injections to the area around the urethra to minimally invasive surgery to more extensive tacking up of the bladder, vagina, and urethra to the pubic bone. Not all of these procedures have been well evaluated, however. I advise you to do your research and to seek a second if not a third opinion if you are considering surgery. The skill of the surgeon, her training, and the technique she recommends can all make a big difference in the outcome. Also, don't forget to ask your surgeon what she considers a surgical success. Some have questionnaires for you to fill out before and after surgery. You list what you want the results to be and then you report on the actual results. Other surgeons use a presurgery test involving a monitor called a urodynamic measurement system. It records how much pressure is needed to open your urethra. The test is repeated after surgery to determine whether or not there is improvement. No procedure is foolproof but many give good results. I wish you the best of luck as you explore your options!

CAUSES OF URGE INCONTINENCE

Urge incontinence compromises your quality of life more than stress incontinence does because you have no control over your bladder and you can't always predict when an accident is about to happen. Sometimes you don't even know you have to go. As one of my patients said, "My bladder has a mind of its own." An accident can happen for no reason or it can be brought on when you wash your hands, have an orgasm, and even just think about urinating.

Some cases can be traced to diabetic nerve disorders or "neuropathy." Unfortunately, however, most women with urge incontinence have no identifiable cause other than aging. There are no office-based diagnostic tests that confirm urge incontinence. The symptoms are so obvious that you just know you have it!

TREATING URGE INCONTINENCE
Medication

Prescription medications can be a great help for some women although these meds are generally costly, must be taken on a continuous basis, and have numerous side effects such as a dry mouth, headaches, fatigue or sleepiness, constipation, and tummy aches. They work by relaxing the smooth muscle of the bladder and blocking certain nerve receptors to the urethra to help keep it closed. That's a positive effect for urge incontinence, yet it's the result of the same "anticholinergic" action of antihistamines and antidepressants that has a negative effect on stress incontinence. However, the medications that are especially for urge incontinence have less of a sedative effect than antihistamines and antidepressants do. Trial and error is the best approach when it comes to medications. Only you

Medications for Urge Incontinence

- Ditropan, Ditropan XL (oxybutynin). This is the original irritable bladder medication. It is prescribed much less often now because it is less effective and has more side effects than newer drugs.
- Detrol, Detrol LA (tolterodine) 1–2 mg twice a day; 2–4 mg daily (Detrol LA)
- Urispas (flavoxate) 100–200 mg three times a day
- Tofranil (imipramine) 10–75 mg nightly or divided up during the day
- Bentyl (dicyclomine) 10–20 mg three times a day. This is a smooth muscle relaxant that has been used for years to treat irritable or spastic colon.
- Levsin (hyoscyamine) 0.375 mg twice daily. This is commonly used to treat irritable bowel syndrome as well.
- Sanctura (trospium) 20 mg twice daily taken on an empty stomach at least 1 hour before meals.
- Vesicare (solifenacin) 5–10 mg daily
- Enablex (darifenacin) 7.5–15 mg daily

can evaluate whether the results are good enough and whether the side effects are tolerable.

Whether you have urge incontinence, stress incontinence, or a urinary tract infection, I want you to do all you can to find solutions and live well with your condition. That's exactly what happened when I treated the patient we met at beginning of this chapter. She took all of my advice to heart. As a result she hasn't had cystitis in over a year and she reports that her sex life is "better than ever." As for me, I got past an initial aversion to doing the Kegel pelvic floor exercises. Once they became a routine part of my life, I felt proud that I had the power to strengthen the muscles that had betrayed me for so long. I hope these success stories will give you the determination and courage to take charge of your urinary troubles and get busy making the changes that can put you back in the mood.

In parts I, II, and III, I taught you about women's health by focusing on the physical—your anatomy, the changes you'll experience over a lifetime, and your potential problems "down there." But, of course, you're a person, not just a body. You have thoughts and emotions that affect your health and well-being. Like most of us these days, you probably have a complex schedule that stresses you out. Finding time to exercise and get enough sleep may be a big challenge for you. Also, even if you know what you should be eating, you may find yourself scarfing down fast food as you go about your busy days. Because I want you to have every possible chance of achieving optimum health for as long as you live, I have devoted part IV to helping you harness the power of the brain-body connection, sidestep its pitfalls, and establish once and for all those "wise lifestyle choices" I keep prescribing.

PART IV

What Happens Down There Doesn't Stay Down There

10

The Female Emotional Response

How a Woman's Brain-Body Connection
Differs from a Man's

IN THIS CHAPTER

- How Stress Affects Your Health

- The Holmes-Rahe Life Stress Inventory Revisited

- Tend and Befriend vs. Fight or Flight

- Stress Relief Strategies That Really Work

Right at the start, I want to state clearly that this chapter is not about serious psychological and emotional disorders such as clinical depression, suicidal ideation, bipolar syndrome, anorexia, bulimia, anxiety, panic attacks, agoraphobia, post-traumatic stress disorder, chemical addictions, or any other condition that should be thoroughly evaluated by mental-health-care providers and treated appropriately.

Unfortunately, that is seldom what happens. A study released in 2008 reported that depression is most often treated by primary care physicians rather than by mental-health-care professionals. What's more, family doctors are often quick to prescribe antidepressants and anti-anxiety drugs. Women are still thought by some doctors to be prone to "hysteria," that old malady with a name that comes from the word for womb. A woman who complains of chest pains may be given a tranquilizer to "calm her nerves" when in fact she has a symptom of heart disease. A man who complains of chest pains gets a cardiac stress test, not a "chill pill"! If your doctor reaches for the prescription pad when he diagnoses you with depression or any other clinical disorder, I urge you to hold off filling the "script" and get a second opinion first.

Even so, women are in fact twice as likely to suffer from depression as men are. Whether this is because of our hormones or our multitasking lives with jobs, kids, husbands, and elderly parents—or a combination of both—is still a matter of debate. For menopausal women, I have found that hormone therapy is often a more appropriate option than mood-altering drugs. For women of all ages, I recommend lifestyle changes wherever possible. However, I am keenly aware that depression can be life-threatening. I monitor and follow up with patients closely and carefully. If they are not improving in short order, I make a referral to a specialist. Psychotropic medication may indeed be called for. However, if you do take drugs, make sure you are getting all the support you need. Antidepressants have powerful side effects and most make you feel "flat." You may no longer feel down but you won't feel up either. Also, watch out for anti-anxiety drugs. They are extremely addictive. A health buddy (see chapter 3) is key here almost more than for any other health problem. Don't go it alone.

HOW STRESS AFFECTS YOUR HEALTH

Having said all that, I'm ready to move on to sharing with you some fascinating findings and healthy strategies for keeping stress at bay. You don't need a doctor to tell you that you have concrete physical reactions to both positive and negative stressful life events. In fact the vernacular is rife with expressions that reflect this fact: "That makes me sick to my stomach". . . "He's a pain in the neck" . . . "It gave me goose bumps". . . "I've got butterflies" . . . "That gave me the chills" . . . "I swallowed hard". . . "I could hardly breathe" . . . "That gave me a headache" . . . "My heart was racing" . . . "I couldn't see straight". . . "Time seemed to stop" . . . "I couldn't think straight" . . . "My cheeks were burning" . . . "My hands were shaking". . . "I got a lump in my throat" . . . "My hair stood on end" . . . "Oh, my aching back!"

You may already know that the internal processes that cause those all-too-familiar sensations can compromise your immune system if stress is unrelenting. Research has shown that the pressures of modern life can be a factor in making us prone to everything from the common cold to cancer. Also, stress can exacerbate autoimmune diseases such as lupus and multiple sclerosis. And certainly the so-called psychosomatic illnesses such as fibromyalgia, vulvodynia, and chronic fatigue syndrome are not "all in your head." "Psych" means mind and "soma" means body. The two are inextricably linked. That's why the symptoms of these conditions are very real. Just as real, of course, are classic complaints including irregular menstrual cycles, frequent upper respiratory problems, rashes, diarrhea, hypertension, high cholesterol, infections, teeth grinding, insomnia, reduced fertility, weight gain..

That's quite a roster! We have to do something about keeping you from falling prey to any of those problems. You know by now that my core mission is to make sure you're in control of your health. Since the very definition of stress is the feeling of being out of control, putting you back in the driver's seat is absolutely crucial to your health and well-being.

To that end, I'll clue you in to a fairly well-kept secret: Women's bodies typically respond to stress in a way that is not at all the same as the way men's bodies respond. In turn, this special feminine reaction makes women have a tendency to behave differently in the face of stress than men do. You can learn to take advantage of what I call your Female Emotional Response and put it to work for you. If you do, you'll go a long way toward minimizing the ill effects of stress in your life. Before I teach you how to do that, though, I want to help you pinpoint the top stressors in your life as a woman. First, I'm going to turn on its ear a long-standing and widely used tool for predicting the likelihood of contracting stress-related illnesses.

THE HOLMES-RAHE LIFE STRESS
INVENTORY REVISITED

Back in 1967 I graduated from high school and left home for the University of Pennsylvania Nursing School—the initial big stressor in my life. That same year a team of psychiatrists named Thomas Holmes and Richard Rahe developed a list of forty-three life events that they deemed to be stressful. They gave each event a number based on just how stressful they thought the event would be. Next they had a grand total of 5,000 patients with various diseases indicate which events had happened to them in the preceding twelve months. By adding up the numbers associated with the events, Holmes and Rahe came up with scores that had a positive correlation to the participants' illnesses. The results were published in the *Journal of Psychosomatic Research* as "The Holmes-Rahe Life Stress Inventory: The Social Readjustment Rating Scale." For a follow-up in 1970, Rahe used the scale in a study of 2,500 sailors and again he came up with a correlation positive enough to suggest a link between stress and disease. In the ensuing decades, the Holmes-Rahe scale has become the gold standard for forecasting who's likely to come down with something as a result of stress.

I'm not in any way refuting the notion that stress and illness are linked. However, I see a serious flaw in the Holmes-Rahe scale. Have a look at the top ten stressors on their list and the numbers that go with them. Keep in mind that the higher the number, the greater the purported impact of the life event:

1. Death of a spouse   100
2. Divorce   73
3. Marital separation from mate   65
4. Detention in jail or other institution   63
5. Death of a close family member   63
6. Major personal injury or illness   53

7.	Marriage	50
8.	Being fired at work	47
9.	Marital reconciliation with mate	45
10.	Retirement from work	45

What is wrong with this picture? You guessed it! Major stressors for women are entirely absent. After all, women were not allowed to serve on Navy ships until 1978. This means that every one of those sailors that Rahe tested in 1970 was a guy. There's no record of whether any of the original 5,000 patients were women, but we do know that there has been a long-standing bias against using female participants in stress studies because of the perceived problems of factoring in hormonal fluctuations due to menstrual cycles. In any case, we can say without a doubt that those sea dogs in Rahe's follow-up study had never been pregnant or given birth or breastfed a baby or gone through menopause. It's also a good bet that not one of them had ever been the major caregiver for a terrible two-year-old, a risk-taking teen, or an elderly parent. And to be really contrarian, would all women of a certain age actually rank death of a spouse and divorce as life's top two stressors with the highest point values? Statistics show that widowers usually remarry but widows by and large do not. To paraphrase sociologist Jessie Bernard, a grande dame of relationship research, men go into marriage with a sense of entitlement while women go into marriage with a sense of obligation. Franz Lehárs's most famous opera isn't called *The Merry Widow* for nothing.

Look, I happen to be married to an absolute gem of a man and for me, the death of my beloved spouse would indeed merit 100 points and be the preeminent life event on the list. I'm just saying in all honesty that the scale, for women as a whole, is skewed from the male perspective. True enough, if you read all forty-three items, you'll find "Pregnancy" at no. 12 with a point score of 40. But please! That score is way too low. Also, no. 14 is "Gaining a new family member" with a score of 39. In parentheses, the researchers put "i.e., birth, adoption, adult moving in, etc." Huh? Just about any woman would break those events out as separate stressors and give them substantial point values. Not only that, but "birth" for a woman isn't just "gaining a new family member." It's giving birth! That's a major life event if there ever were one. And for women who want to conceive but can't, that disappointment is perhaps the biggest stressor of their lives.

Moving right along, no. 23 at a paltry 29 points is "Son or daughter leaving home." In parentheses the researchers explain that this includes "marriage, attending college, joined military." Wait a minute! Welcoming a son-in-law or daughter-in-law and moving your kid into a college dorm are the precise emotional equivalents of having your child possibly deployed to a war zone? I don't think so! Also note, ranking "Detention in jail or other institution" as no. 4 on the list with a point value of 63 ignores the fact that historically many more men than women are incarcerated. The 2007 data from the United Stated Bureau of Justice, the most recent available, show that 86 percent of prisoners were male and only 14 percent were female.

The full Holmes-Rahe scale does include some events that apparently aren't gender-specific, such as financial problems, sexual difficulties, troubles with in-laws, and celebrating major holidays. But what about miscarriages, abortions, leaving the baby in day care, or being a stay-at-home mom? I remember crying every day after having twins when my firstborn was only fifteen months old and still in diapers with a bottle. And what about dealing with boomerang kids, being a trailing spouse when a husband gets transferred, caring for a special-needs child, or having a sick or elderly parent move in? This last one is extremely common and it is a huge stressor that almost always falls to women. My family is a case in point. My sister Eileen cared for my late mother during a long illness and is now caring for my father.

I could also argue that even the issues that appear to be gender-neutral truly are not. "Financial problems" for a man could mean a layoff and for a woman that could mean the old saw about "marrying him for life but not for lunch" along with her own job pressures. "Sexual difficulties" for a husband could be erectile dysfunction and maybe an enlarged prostate, while for a woman that could mean dealing with his often futile attempts at intercourse and his accompanying bruised ego while she is also coping with her own vaginal atrophy. "Trouble with in-laws" is almost always code for wife/mother-in-law conflicts when the guys spend the whole visit watching the game while the women lob not-so-subtle attacks at one another about everything from recipes to mopping the kitchen floor to whether the kids should be allowed to have candy. Finally we come to "Celebrating the major holidays." Holmes and Rahe rated that one at a measly 12 points. But guess who still does most of the shopping, wrapping, decorating, cooking, and cleaning even though it's been three decades since the concept of "role-free marriages" was first floated by neo-feminists? Answer: The wife—the very same person who makes sure there are fresh towels in the guest bathroom and just-laundered sheets on the guest beds. Some things never change from generation to generation! I am typically the one on duty for my huge extended family for Thanksgiving. That means leaves in the table, linens, special glasses cleaned, decorations, buying tons of food for the long weekend, and on and on. I'm stressed out just thinking about it!

Interestingly, a version of Holmes-Rahe has been created for use with children and teens although no version has ever been made for women. However, while the list for young people includes such events as birth of a sibling, parents' divorce, failing a grade in school, and beginning to date, it does not include "Getting your first period." The girls are ignored just as women are ignored in the adult scale.

And so? I suggest that you simply make your own list! You know better than anyone what your strictly female stressors are, depending where you are in the feminine life cycle right now. Writing them down will help you be alert to possible problems. For the record, a quick infor-mal poll of my female patients elicited the following additions to the stressor list, in no particular order.

- Got a new puppy. I was the one who had to housebreak him and I walk him and clean up after him even though my husband and I both work.
- Pumped breast milk for six months in the lactation room at the office.
- Planned my wedding.
- Lost weight before I went to my twentieth high school reunion.
- Lost weight so I could look decent as the mother-of-the-bride.
- Put my mother in a nursing home.
- Found out my husband has been cheating on me.
- Found out my husband has been going to a prostitute—or as they like to call themselves so the stigma seems less for the guy (and the girl I suppose), "escorts"
- Started helping my daughter out by babysitting my grandchildren while she works.
- Got bad news on amniocentesis but kept the Down syndrome baby even though we said we wouldn't
- Baby born with spina bifida
- Stillborn baby, full-term. (My milk came in even though I took something to stop it.)
- Preemie died after two weeks in the NICU
- Weaned my baby
- Husband had prostate surgery and now wears diapers and can't get it up
- Custody battle and now I have to leave my kids with him and the other woman every weekend
- Went through my mother's things after she died. (My brother didn't help at all.)
- Had my parents and his parents here for Christmas when the baby was only three months old
- The first time I wasn't the one to cook Thanksgiving dinner. I was a guest at my daughter's table. I felt like I'd been put out to pasture!

- The dog died. This was right after my last child left for college.
- My daughter lost the baby.
- My daughter has been trying IVF but it's not working.
- I found out my tubes are blocked so us not getting pregnant is my fault.

Those stressors are all so true and sad. I hope you can freely think of stressors in the last year that merit being on your personal list. Fortunately, as I mentioned earlier, recent research has at last shed light on what happens to our feminine inner circuitry when we're stressed. The study also shows how we typically behave under stress and how we can turn that response into a positive one. Now we have one more way to show for certain that we're not just "small men"!

TEND AND BEFRIEND VS. FIGHT OR FLIGHT

Unless you've been living on Mars, you've surely heard by now about the "fight or flight" reaction to stress. The term was coined in 1915 by Harvard physiologist Walter Cannon to describe the body's response to perils, whether perceived or actual. The Hungarian-born endocrinologist Han Selye expanded on this idea beginning in 1936 by calling bad stress by the term "distress" (e.g., getting fired, having to foreclose on your home, being injured) and good stress by the term "eustress" (e.g., getting married, winning the lottery, having a baby). He pointed out that both distress and eustress cause the "fight or flight" response. As a quick recap, we share this primitive predilection with other animals, as did our long-ago ancestors for whom impending danger could easily have been an approaching tiger with teeth bared rather than a performance review at work or a traffic jam when you're late to pick up your kid at day care. The magnitude of the body's involuntary response, with the brain's hypothalamic-pituitary axis (HPA) sending a system-wide Code Red, made sense when the emergency really was an imminent attack by a tiger. The HPA triggers the firing of neurons and a flood of hormones. For Mr. and Mrs. Neanderthal, the fact that adrenaline and cortisol, among other hormones, created a hyper-alert state with glucose as a ready energy supply was definitely advantageous. So was the accompanying shut-down of temporarily unnecessary functions such as digestion and sexual response. With all available resources marshaled for defense or retreat, early humans were all set either to club the tiger or head for the hills at breakneck speed.

For us, though, the likelihood of the actual need to fight or flee is fairly remote. Unless you happen to step into the path of a speeding vehicle or encounter a mugger on a dark and stormy night, you're most often going to be all revved up for a heroic battle or a high-speed get-away when all you can do is meekly acquiesce to an angry boss or text the day-care center to let them know you're stuck on the expressway.

Another cause of stress early in human history (and sadly, still in some countries today) was the feast-or-famine cycle. As a result, we developed the "thrifty gene" that creates and holds onto fat stores for use when the food supply is low. Most of us don't need that extra fuel any longer but we pack on belly fat from excess cortisol during stress anyway. (See chapter 11 for more on belly fat.)

Suppressing the fight-or-flight response can have unhealthy consequences. This is especially true if you are pretty much always at least somewhat stressed. Your adrenal glands get depleted, the extra cortisol contributes to belly fat, your blood pressure stays too high, your immune system doesn't do its job well, your digestive tract gets out of whack, and your reproductive system can go haywire. Yet while we can't eliminate our twenty-first-century varieties of stress altogether—there will always be performance reviews and traffic jams—what we can do is tune in to our uniquely female ability to counter the ill effects.

The secret weapon we have is a hormone called oxytocin, the same one that floods the body of a birthing woman and motivates people toward what sociologists call "pair bonding." Men produce oxytocin, too, but in much smaller quantities than we do. Not only that, but their oxytocin has the formidable task of tamping down the anger and aggressiveness that testosterone can inspire. Our oxytocin, on the other hand, teams up with estrogen to create a stress paradigm that UCLA researchers headed by Shelly Taylor, Ph.D., dubbed "Tend and Befriend" in 2000. This translates into our powerful instinct to nurture our children and our proclivity to form close ties with other women.

In one classic example of the difference between males and females when it comes to handling modern-day stress, men who have a bad day at work often isolate themselves and self-medicate. In other words, when they get home they only want to plunk down in front of the television with a beer. They may even take out their frustrations on the family by snapping at the wife and kids. In contrast, a woman who comes home after a stressful stint at the office usually welcomes the chance to be with her kids. Mothering becomes an antidote to career pressures and a reminder of what really matters in her life. She may also call her own mother or her sister or a girlfriend to vent and get support. Beyond that, she may look for a way to reach out to someone who is worse off than she is—an elderly aunt living alone or a new neighbor who left her friends and family behind when she moved to town. This is what I mean by the Female Emotional Response. And even if a woman wants to be all alone at times, as I often did when returning from my busy practice to three babies, the truth is women feel too guilty to indulge in solitude. I remember when our kids were small that my doctor husband could simply ignore their cries and their tugging on his pant leg while he was on the phone with sick patients. I never could do that.

STRESS RELIEF STRATEGIES
THAT REALLY WORK

I help my patients counter stress in ways that may seem counterintuitive if you're thinking only about the fight-or-flight model. For example, I don't necessarily recommend a long soak alone in a bubble bath. (For one thing, the perfumed bubbles could bring on allergic vaginitis. But that's another story!) The bubble bath remedy is a time-honored stress buster but it actually amounts to a type of "flight" by isolating you from others. As a woman, that may be precisely the wrong move.

Yes, busy working mothers in particular do need occasional "alone time." However, in most cases you're better off baking cookies with the kids instead of sequestering yourself behind a closed bathroom door while they occupy themselves with homework or video games. When you share some cozy kitchen time with your children, you'll stimulate the release of the love hormone, oxytocin, and give it a chance to enhance the effects of estrogen. Your husband should only be so lucky! The poor guy may get some benefit by hitting balls in the backyard with the boys but only because the physical activity "lets off steam." He doesn't have that inner female cocktail of oxytocin and estrogen to soothe his frayed nerves and make workday pressures recede. But you do! Just make sure you activate it by calling into play your tend-and-befriend response.

To help you do that, try Dr. Marie's De-Stress Dozen—my twelve tips to keep you on an even keel when stress threatens to push you off balance:

1. Volunteer. There's really nothing like doing good to help you do well! I know you're busy, but even a few hours a month reading to the blind or helping out at a local food bank can be remarkably restorative for your body and soul. It seems that the busier you are, the more likely you are to give of your free time. I have always agreed to serve on committees and on nonprofit boards when asked—especially if the organizations promoted the welfare and interests of disadvantaged women. Another idea: Why not volunteer to be a health buddy for an elderly neighbor or friend newly diagnosed with cancer or a chronic illness?

2. Join a club. Study after study has shown that the more socially connected we are, the better we feel. Face time is what

counts, not Facebook time. Get away from that computer and make some flesh-and-blood female friends who share your interests! A book club, a gardening club, a dining club, a theater and movie club—any or all of these will boost your morale and your immune system.

3. Meet your girlfriends for lunch. Eating at your desk or on the run is a risky habit. Get out of the office at least a couple of times a week to meet a female confidante. Or form a neighborhood play group that gives each mom an afternoon off on a rotating basis. Use your free-from-toddlers time to get together with a woman who has a sympathetic ear.

4. Take the kids to the park. Even if you have a big backyard of your own, seek out the social setting of a neighborhood playground. The kids will benefit from some sandbox-and-jungle-gym time, and you'll get a chance to bond with other mothers. Just what the doctor ordered!

5. Get the kids involved in the kitchen. So what if they make a mess? Many hands make light work and the children will learn math skills by measuring, plus have fun mixing and mashing. Good therapy for one and all!

6. Borrow a child. If you don't have a kid of your own handy, sign up to take an orphan to the zoo or let your neighbors know you're available for an occasional babysitting stint. Being the unofficial "aunt" in a young person's life is a win-win situation.

7. Send good wishes for any reason or no reason at all. This absolutely works. On a day when you're frazzled and pressured and totally on circuit overload, dash off a quick e-mail of good cheer to someone you care about. What goes around comes around—and that includes goodwill!

8. Ask directions. I'm serious. The tend-and-befriend researchers found that the old saw about men not asking for

directions is no joke. A guy's testosterone-fed stoicism really does keep him from soliciting help from others. You, on the other hand, can get that oxytocin-estrogen mix pumping by letting people know you need guidance—whether it's about how to reach an actual destination or an emotional one!

9. Support the man in your life. Speaking of guys, since the man in your life is hard-wired to hide in his cave when he's feeling down, you need to find a way to touch him both literally and figuratively. If your effort ends up turning him on, so much the better. As we saw in chapter 2, sex is one of nature's very best uppers for both of you!

10. Laugh with those you love. Humor really is the best medicine. Moping all by yourself is bad medicine, but getting together with friends and family to share a few laughs is a potent stress reliever. Rent a funny movie, watch Comedy Central, or get out to a comedy club now and then. You'll feel the tension drain away.

11. Try a little retail therapy. Spending money is definitely not the point. That will only make you feel guilty. My version of retail therapy is all about the fun of shopping, especially with the women in your life. Don't go on an impulse shopping spree all by yourself. Also, shopping online simply does not count! What works is to get your girlfriend or your mother or your daughter or your sister to join you on a bargain-hunting jaunt. The pleasure in this strategy is not so much in making purchases as it is in the browsing and the camaraderie. Sharing the dressing room with a friend while trying on clothes is a hoot! Go ahead and treat yourself to a few well-chosen baubles but as with everything in life, moderation is the key!

12. Exercise with friends and family. Double the benefit of physical activity by getting some connection time with

Dr. Marie's Three C's for Stress Relief

Control. If stress is the feeling of being out of control, then the obvious antidote is to do everything within your power to regain at least some control.

- If you have been diagnosed with a life-threatening or chronic illness, go into action. Research your disease so that you know all of your treatment options and can knowledgeably participate in your care. Find support groups, perhaps an actual one along with one in cyberspace where anonymity fosters frankness. Also, face up to the task of making contingency plans such as arranging for the care of your children if you should have to go to the hospital. Be sure to go over your finances to see where you really stand.

- If you are stuck in a job with a monster of a boss, consider every possible exit strategy. Look for new jobs on Internet job boards and social networks. Think about becoming an entrepreneur if you've always wanted to turn your greenhouse hobby or talent for knitting into a business. Learn the laws for running a business in your state. Join a group for female small-business owners. Oddly, even if you remain mired in your miserable "day job," the simple act of *trying* to get control will help.

- The same is true if your marriage is dragging you down. Don't put up a facade for the world. Go to the family counselor at your church. Confide in your girlfriends. Call your sister. Again, just reaching out for help will give you at least some sense of being in control.

Change. Analyze your life. Are you repeating the same destructive patterns over and over again? Are you in a rut—or more than one rut? When somebody asks how you are, is the answer, "Same ol', same ol'"? Make a promise to yourself that you will find fresh goals, seek new friends, freshen up your outlook, and otherwise infuse your existence with excitement and energy. Even little changes such as a new hairstyle, trying an ethnic cuisine for the first time, or rearranging the living room furniture can make a difference. Big changes will make an even bigger difference. This is your life. As the saying goes, it's not a dress rehearsal!

Connect. And now we've come full circle back to the Female Emotional Response that makes you want to "tend and befriend." Nurture others and you will nurture your own soul as well. Be part of a caring support network and you won't fall very far before your loved ones catch you and lift you up again. You need them, and they need you. Don't miss out on the best stress buster a woman can have!

others in the bargain. Join a mall walking group or sign up for salsa lessons or go biking with the kids. If you can get your guy involved in any of this, that would be good for both of you!

Feeling better? I thought so! By "tending and befriending," you have regained a sense of control in your life. The ability to touch the lives of others for the better and also to let people help you are sources of emotional and physical well-being that we should tap into again and again. Not only that, but by taming the stress monster, you are already on your way to curbing excess cortisol and therefore trimming the circumference of your waist. This is the single most important step you can take to ensure that you will maintain your good health as the years go by. In the next chapter I'll not only tell you why that's true, but I'll give you all the help and encouragement you need to achieve an ideal WHR. What's that? Read on to find out!

11

Waist Management

Winning the War against Womanly Weight Gain

> **IN THIS CHAPTER**
> - Know Your Waist-Hip Ratio (WHR)
> - All Fat Is Not Created Equal
> - Shape Shifts during a Woman's Life

Throughout this book you've learned that modern medicine has an impressive array of sophisticated diagnostic tools and tests. They all have their place. Yet when it comes to assessing your risk of everything from heart disease to diabetes to breast and colon cancer, all you need is a household item that's probably already in your sewing kit or your desk drawer: a cloth tape measure.

The circumference of your waist is one of the single most accurate predictors of the future status of your health. I have been writing and speaking about this topic for some time after observing it during my many years in practice. Recent studies from around the world have corroborated my findings and I continue to be quoted as a leading expert on the subject.

Taking the test a step further, if you divide your waist measurement by the circumference of your hips, you'll get an even more precise take on what your chances are of staying well down the road. The best news of all, however, is that should this simple little exercise in long division put you on notice for possible problems, you can make a mid-course correction just by paring even *one inch* off your waistline. And if you can lose two inches, so much the better. This rule holds true *no matter how much you weigh now.* What follows is everything you need to know to calculate your waist-hip ratio (WHR) correctly and make a lifetime commitment to keeping it within the ideal range.

KNOW YOUR WAIST-HIP RATIO (WHR)

The first step is to measure your waist *at the smallest point*—that is, where your waistband or a belt would go. I realize that if you've packed on a few too many pounds and/or you have an "apple" shape (see page 319), you may not have a "smallest" point. In that case, find the bottom of your rib cage and measure that area.

Many sources, including the Centers for Disease Control and Prevention, suggest that you should measure around the area where your belly button is, but that is not as accurate. Most of us who have been pregnant one or more times have a "pooch" of stretched skin with some fat. However, it's not the kind of fat we're trying to locate. See the following pages for a full explanation of the two kinds of body fat. For now, though, trust me. Measuring your "pooch" is not what you want to do. (Men actually can get an accurate measure around the belly button area.)

Don't cheat yourself out of a true measurement by sucking in your gut or pulling the tape measure tight enough to indent your flesh. The idea is to face once and for all exactly how many inches around your abdomen really is. Nobody has to know this information except you! Seriously, not even your doctor is likely to find out. The value of WHR is well known by physicians but the majority of them still don't whip out a tape measure during your annual physical and keep track of the results year by year. They continue to rely on your weight and height although those numbers fall far short of your WHR as a health indicator.

For the record, the highly touted body mass index (BMI) is also less reliable than WHR because results vary widely depending on how much muscle mass people have in relation to fat. My mantra is "It's not how much you weigh, but where you weigh it." Of course, it's possible to find out what percentage of body fat you have, but the only true tests involve being submerged underwater or using calipers. The home scales that purport to tell you how much body fat you have give iffy results. Why bother with any of this when your trusty tape measure will tell all? True, if you are obese with a BMI of thirty or more, knowing your waist circumference won't add much new information, but for women who are overweight or normal weight, waist circumference and WHR are the most important measures. You may be what is popularly called "skinny fat." That is, your body weight is fine but your health risks are high because you have excess visceral fat in your abdomen around your organs. You may not even see it but your waist measurement will let you know about it.

Once you've measured your waist at the right spot, measure your hips at the widest place. Now do the math: waist divided by hips. Consider using a spreadsheet on your computer if you know how to do that. You can put the waist measurement in one cell, the hip measurement in another cell, and create a division function in a third cell. Then every time you want to check up on yourself for progress or mainte- nance, you can just copy your formula, paste it into adjacent cells, and enter the new numbers if any. But whether you get as geeky as that or simply use a calculator or a pencil and paper, you're hoping to see the following:

- a waist size of thirty-five inches or lower
- a WHR of .8 or lower

ALL FAT IS NOT CREATED EQUAL

Back when I was in medical school and first saw drawings of typical fat distribution patterns in males and females, I felt oddly offended

by the artist's rendering of what my girlfriends and I had always rue-
fully referred to as our "saddlebags." I've never been overweight
but I had always wished my hips and thighs were a little less ample.
Those sketches of women compared to men in the anatomy textbook
seemed at first to be an unfair exaggeration of a bottom-heavy feminine form.

I was also surprised to learn that about 25 percent of the body of a
healthy man of normal weight is made of fat, while a whopping one-
third of the body of a healthy woman of normal weight is fat. However,
in short order I found out that the kind of fat carried by fertile women
is actually protective. Our saddlebags are good for us! On the other
hand, the fat storehouse for men is the belly. This so-called "visceral
fat" is a health risk. As we'll see when I explain the changes we women
go through over the years, females are also prone to visceral fat at various stages in their lives. That's why I went to so much trouble earlier to
educate you about the importance of a good WHR.

Here's how our two types of body fat differ:

- Subcutaneous fat, meaning "under the skin," is inactive. It's
  largely found on your legs and backside even if you're lean. This
  fat is nothing but padding and potential fuel. Nature, thanks to
  the effects of estrogen, gives us a good supply to draw on during
  pregnancy and breastfeeding. Men have some subcutaneous fat,
  too, of course, but not nearly as much as we do.
- Visceral fat collects deep inside the abdomen around your organs.
  It is in fact an organ itself in that it behaves as an endocrine
  gland like your thyroid or your pituitary. This type of adipose
  tissue secretes hormones that help regulate metabolism, but that
  positive function is offset by the fact that belly fat also produces
  molecules called cytokines. They promote inflammation and
  increase the likelihood of the development of a long list of
  diseases, many of them life-threatening or at best chronic.

You can't eliminate visceral fat with any of the popular procedures peddled by plastic surgeons. A "mommy makeover" with a tummy tuck and a breast lift only involves getting rid of excess stretched skin after pregnancy and breastfeeding. Liposuction can draw out some of your subcutaneous fat but it won't touch the dangerous stuff that's inside.

Also, please don't fall for the fad called "colonic cleansing"! Whether you take the powerful over-the-counter laxatives advertised for this purpose or you go to a pricey "colonic hydrotherapist" for a "high enema," you will *not* lose belly fat. You will also not be any more "detoxified" or "purified" or "irrigated" than you will be if you eat a high-fiber diet and establish regular bowel habits (see chapter 8). Besides that, a "high colonic" could flush out important electrolytes and perforate your colon with serious consequences including infection.

So what's the answer? Subcutaneous fat is stubborn, as though nature won't let you part with the ready stash that's meant for child-bearing. Yet your body gladly gives up belly fat even if all you do is add a mere thirty minutes of walking to your daily routine. A study done at Duke University in 2004 called STRRIDE (Studies of Targeted Risk Reduction Interventions through Defined Exercise) showed that people who walked for a half an hour a day, six days a week, lost significant amounts of belly fat as revealed by CT scans after eight months. Also, the control group that did no exercise showed an increase in belly fat of 8.6 percent even though their average weight gain was only 1 percent. The participants in the study were told not to change their diets in any way. In other words, the walking group lost hazardous visceral fat with exercise alone. We can only imagine how much more they could have lost if they had modified their calorie intake. As I have said for a long time, exercise is king and diet is queen. Now, though, I've started saying that sleep is the overlord of the world! A recent study showed that lack of sleep cancels out the beneficial effect of exercise. Another study showed that not getting adequate sleep contributes to weight gain.

Now let's have a look at how our female predisposition to belly fat alters over our life cycle. In earlier chapters, we've talked about the Triple Goddess theme that runs through the history of so many societies and cultures. Taking that mythical or religious concept into the realm of science, we've also explored the differences in our bodies during the three seasons of our adult lives beginning with the menarche and moving on to fertility and then menopause. Yet in a very real sense, a woman has several different bodies over a lifetime: the prepubertal body of childhood, the fertile body of the childbearing years, the pregnant body if she conceives, the postpartum body with or without the breastfeeding component, the perimenopausal body, and the postmenopausal body. All of these versions of herself are distinct hormonally and in terms of fat distribution. Being informed about the inevitable variations can help us counter any ill effects and keep the WHR where it should be.

SHAPE SHIFTS DURING A WOMAN'S LIFE

You've probably heard by now about the body shape classifications that have been labeled "apples,"and "pears." Women who are apple-shaped have their highest concentration of fat in the abdominal area while women who are pear-shaped carry their weight in the hips, thighs, and buttocks. There are sub-categories such as string beans and bananas who have straight bodies but are actually apples for medical purposes. There is also an inverted pear with a generous bosom and small hips who is classified medically as an apple. Finally the hourglass figure is a type of pear. These are the key points to remember:

- Most women during the fertile years are pears with weight concentrated on their hips and thighs. This is protective subcutaneous fat.
- Some women, because of their balance of hormones, have apple body types even during the fertile years. Unlike men, they do

have substantial pear zone fat but they add belly fat just as men do when they gain weight.

- Women who are string beans or bananas are not prone to holding on to fat stores in any particular area. Because of their hormone balance, however, if they gain weight it will usually go to the apple zone.

Males remain apples from childhood right on through old age. Females—whether they are predominantly apple, pears, or string beans—undergo a series of transformations as follows:

CHILDHOOD

Little girls are apples just like little boys. Have a look the next time you're at the beach or a swimming pool and you'll see that all the kids have rounded tummies. Unfortunately though, too many children are packing on excess belly fat these days. Childhood obesity is nothing less than an epidemic. Consequently, youngsters are contracting diseases such as diabetes 2 that were once the province of adults.

Also, if a young girl picks up belly fat and carries it with her into puberty, she'll end up with both apple fat and pear fat. That will increase her percentage of overall fat to an unacceptable level. Parents and schools need to make a concerted effort to get kids up off the couch and out from in front of computer games. They also need to teach kids good nutrition right from the start and not let them exist on fast food, sweets, and sodas—even so-called diet sodas, which can actually promote belly fat! And for kids, inadequate sleep is linked to packing on the fat just as it is in adults! If there are little girls in your life—or little boys for that matter— do your part to help them keep their apple tendencies under control.

PUBERTY

A friend of mine who teaches at a summer camp says that she never ceases to be amazed each July when the girls she said goodbye to the previous August as "tweens" come back as teenagers who already look like women. Typically when a girl is somewhere between the ages of twelve and fourteen, hormones kick in and direct most of the fat that she gains to settle on her hips and thighs, and also her breasts. A sudden growth spurt plus the menarche go along with this. The girl seems transformed practically overnight! No wonder we have self-esteem issues at that confusing juncture in our lives. Nothing in the closet fits any more, we're a head taller than the boys in our class, we're dealing with a monthly flow, and our thighs jiggle in gym class!

If you're a teen right now, don't try to ease this transition by indulging in sweets and other high-calorie snacks. You probably are hungrier than you've ever been, but stick with healthy choices such as fruits, vegetables, whole grains, cheese, and fish. Also, watch out for eating disorders! You're setting yourself up for a lifetime of health problems from infertility to osteoporosis if you try to emulate the über-skinny models and actresses you see on magazine covers and in the movies. In addition, one theory holds that young teens fall into anorexia and bulimia because they want to get rid of the fleshy breasts and hips that mean they're growing up and away from childhood. Another cause of eating disorders can be extreme perfectionism—the desire to keep being "the best little girl in the world." If you or a teen you love seems to be heading for an eating disorder, please get help.

Remember, though, that not all thin girls and women are eating disordered. No two women are exactly alike. Each of us has a balance of hormones that plays a part in our individual body shapes:

- Most of us are pears with breast measurements at least somewhat smaller than hip measurements and more fat in the pear zone than the apple zone.
- Maybe, though, you have an "hourglass figure" with full breasts and hips defined by a wasp waist. That means you are estrogen

dominant. That is, the balance of estrogen and androgen is tipped fully toward estrogen.

- If you're a string bean or a banana, you have boyishly slim hips and small breasts. You also have a tendency to add belly fat. This is because your balance of estrogen and androgen is tipped toward androgens including testosterone. You may also be prone to polycystic ovary syndrome (PCOS) a disorder that is characterized by fertility problems and by androgenic symptoms such as the growth of facial hair. See chapter 7 for complete information. Also, many girls with PCOS have mild obesity and insulin resistance and are at risk of becoming the so called "skinny fat" type.
- If you tend to gain weight around your middle even during the fertile years, you are an apple with more testosterone than average. Some apples can develop PCOS.

PREGNANCY

During pregnancy you experience rapid and profound changes in hormone production with estradiol bathing the fetus and progesterone continuing to pump instead of pausing as it does when you have your period. You also stop making corticotropin-releasing hormone (CRH), a stress hormone, because the placenta takes over that job. Your breasts enlarge and, of course, your uterus expands as the fetus grows. Your hips widen as the ligaments relax to allow the pelvis to permit passage of the baby down the birth canal and out into the world. Most women gain between seventeen and forty pounds during pregnancy depending on pre-pregnancy weight. Women may gain even more if they're carrying twins or other multiples. You are "eating for two" (or three or four!) so you'll be hungrier than normal, but don't overdo it. Gaining more weight than you and the baby or babies need will put you at risk for gestational diabetes and other problems. Also, you'll have more "baby fat" to contend with after the birth. During pregnancy our body fat is shifting. We are drawing from our pear zone stores and if we take in more calories than necessary, we store the excess in our bellies—the apple zone.

POSTPARTUM

In a scene from the classic film *Gone With the Wind* that takes place after the birth of Scarlett O'Hara's first child, Mammy is tugging on the laces of Scarlett's corset. They have this exchange about Scarlett's waist:

> **Scarlett:** *Mammy, you've just got to make it 18½ again.*
>
> **Mammy:** *You done had a baby Miss Scarlett. You ain't never gonna be no 18½ again.*

Mammy was almost certainly correct. Pregnancy does indeed usually add inches around the middle. One study showed that the average woman gains seven pounds with each successive pregnancy. Because of hormone shifts, most of the excess *avoirdupois* will be deposited in the apple zone as belly fat. This is the beginning of a woman's transition over the years from pear to apple. However, I'll say this now and I'll emphasize it again later: You won't gain belly fat if you don't gain too much weight! Belly fat is not inevitable—not for men and not for women. All that's inevitable is the body's inclination to store *extra* weight in the apple zone.

You may also be at risk for postpartum depression and that could cause you either to eat too much to ease the emotional pain or eat too little out of listlessness and loss of joy in life. One theory that resulted from a study by a team of researchers at the National Institutes of Health showed that sudden cessation of the production of CRH by the placenta may play a part in the symptoms of postpartum depression. Your own body may be taking a while to start making CRH again and that can cause a spectrum of feelings ranging from sadness to severe depression. Even so, as a doctor and as a mother who had twins when my firstborn

Can Hormone Therapy Help with Weight Control?

Apparently the answer is yes. Results of the Postmenopausal Estrogen/Progestin Interventions (PEPI) Trial and other observational studies showed that women who take HT preserve their WHR, gain less weight, and have better balance because of preserved muscle strength. Also, research in animals published by the American Chemical Society in 2007 showed how estrogen receptors located in the hypothalamus serve as a master switch to control food intake, energy use, and body fat distribution. When the special receptors were destroyed, the animals immediately began to eat more food, burn less energy, and gain weight. And, yes, the weight went totally to the middle in the form of excess visceral fat. The animals also developed an impaired tolerance to glucose, which set them up for metabolic syndrome and diabetes 2. Low-dose HT may help keep postmenopausal women from having these same problems. (See chapter 6 to find out whether HT is safe for you to take.)

was fifteen months old, I have to add that sleep deprivation is a huge factor in postpartum emotional problems. Study after study has shown that lack of sleep contributes to stress, and stress makes you produce lots of cortisol. This in turn promotes the storing of visceral fat. Steal a few winks when the baby is sleeping even if that means letting the dishes pile up or the birth announcements sit on your desk. Everything else can wait. You need your sleep!

BREASTFEEDING

As I mentioned in chapter 5, when you're nursing a baby, your body is in a kind of temporary menopause. You're probably not ovulating and your estrogen production is on the low side. That tips the balance toward testosterone, which means an increased tendency toward belly fat. In defense you need to eat wisely, take long walks pushing the baby in the stroller, get down on the floor for some Mommy and Me exercises during the baby's tummy time—and once again, get enough sleep!

PERIMENOPAUSE

As your supply of estrogen begins to dwindle, usually in your midforties, you continue the process that will take you full cycle from the fertile pear years back to the apple shape you shared with males when you were a child. Nature seems to know we no longer have a need for the pear zone fat on our hips and thighs, so one aesthetically pleasing result during this transition in our lives is that our backsides and our legs slim down. You may be surprised to find that you can now fit into skinny jeans—as long as the waist is low-rise. You've probably picked up a "muffin top" even as you lost your saddle bags. This is what we used to call "middle-age spread." However—and here I go again—if you keep extra weight at bay, you won't have much if any dreaded belly fat!

POSTMENOPAUSE

After menopause when estrogen production by the ovaries has stopped, all women begin storing excess fat in their middles. The irony is that belly fat itself produces a form of estrogen but since progesterone production has completely ceased, this estrogen is "unopposed." That's not good! It means an increase in the risk of breast cancer and endometrial cancer risk. In addition, much of the increased fat store incites the release of cortisol, the stress hormone that can cause all sorts of physical and emotional ills. (See chapter 10 for more on this topic.) However, can you find the key word in the first sentence of this paragraph that lets you know "middle-age spread" is not a given? Ah hah! That's right. The word is "excess." If you keep your weight, and more specifically

Dr. Marie's Four "Fs" for Fighting Belly Fat: Fiber, Fat, Fitness, and Fluids

1. **Fiber** foods. High fiber, unprocessed, plant-based foods (fruits, vegetables, nuts, and grains) are chock-full of antioxidants and phytochemicals and they slow down the dangerous glycemic or insulin response to sugar, sweets, and white flour foods.

2. **Fat.** Healthy omega-3s are plentiful in grass-fed animals, cold-water fish, flax seed, and nuts. They boost your brain and heart health, reduce inflammation, and help just about every cell in your body.

3. **Fitness.** Exercise for your body and spirit. This may include Smart Sex, too. You'll shrink your waist size and banish stress all at the same time—and sleep better to boot.

4. **Fluids.** Lots of water is great. Coffee in moderation is okay as well as one alcoholic drink a day. Juice is good, too. Avoid sodas, however—those with sugar as well as those with artificial sweeteners. Up to one glass of wine is good but more is not. Alcohol is good for heart health and insulin in small doses and bad for breasts, blood pressure, and waist line in larger doses. Both kinds promote weight and waist gain.

your waist circumference, under control you don't have to end up with a "meno-pot" of any consequence! Incidentally, your metabolism doesn't slow down perceptibly with age unless you do! If you're no longer running in circles taking care of kids, doing copious loads of laundry, and cooking family meals, you're probably expending less energy these days. The solution is to add regular exercise to your routine to make up for the lost schlepping factor. Exercise not only helps you lose belly fat but it also builds lean muscle mass. Muscle is a fat-burning machine that works even when you're sleeping. Eating right helps too, of course!

See the sidebar for my easy-to-remember formula for lifelong "waist management." Follow it whether you're an apple, a pear, or a string bean, and no matter where you are in the female life cycle:

That brings us almost to the end of our intimate "office visit." As I said in the very first pages of this book, my hope is that you'll come back again and again to reread passages that can help you live well with your woman's body, mind, and soul all the years of your life. Yet before I sign off, I want to leave you with a message about your health care that comes straight from my heart. You'll find it when you turn the page. . . .

Afterword

Dr. Marie's "Lifestyle Pill"

Remember back on the very first page of this book when I asked you to imagine that you could step into my office for a consultation? Now our visit is almost over. Yet before you leave I'm going to write a prescription for you. You don't have to take it to a pharmacy or pay a single cent to get it filled. You've heard me mention it before: my Lifestyle Pill. It's not easy to "swallow" but it can reduce your risk of cancer, heart disease, diabetes, osteoporosis, stroke, liver disease, kidney disease, and a host of other ailments by an amazing 80 percent or more. Not only that, but your odds of living to a ripe old age with your faculties and physical functions intact will rise dramatically.

The residents of Okinawa in Japan know this all too well. They've been consuming the Lifestyle Pill for years and they have the largest population of centenarians in the world. What's more, 80 percent of Okinawa's elderly live independently with no need for hospitalization or nursing home care. Their diet consists largely of locally grown plants including soy. They lead active yet relatively stress-free lives. In their small villages, they enjoy the comfort and support of friends, family, and the community as a whole. Sadly, however, studies have shown that younger Okinawans are beginning to emulate our American lifestyle. As a result, obesity, disease, and untimely death are on the rise.

The message is clear. For many Americans, their way of life is dangerous to their health. They rely on fast food that has huge numbers of calories yet has nutrients processed out of it. Even when they cook their own food, they are partial to red meat, white bread, and sweets. They drink copious amounts of soda, whether sugary or artificially sweetened. They multitask and subject themselves to nearly constant stress. They don't get regular exercise, take time for nurturing relationships and sex, or get nearly enough sleep. Many of them smoke and drink too much alcohol.

But you're not among that number, right? You've read this book. You now know that if you kick destructive habits and embrace a new set of behaviors, you'll be doing wonders for your physical, emotional, and spiritual health. Naturally, you'll also take advantage of what modern medicine has to offer when the need arises. Even so, if you're as healthy as possible to begin with, then everything from medication to surgery will go better for you than it would if your well-being were compromised by unhealthy lifestyle choices.

There is talk now about the possibility in the not-so-distant future of personalized medicine utilizing information from our genes to predict the best prevention and treatments for each of us individually. Yet the pie-in-the-sky promise of a genomic crystal ball belies the fact that we already know how to prevent the major causes of mortality: swallowing the Lifestyle Pill.

I want to leave you with the hope and assurance that the power to have the most optimal health possible is in your own hands. No one can take that away from you. Here, as a refresher to carry with you as you go, is the list of ingredients in the Lifestyle Pill:

- Trust yourself. You know more than you think you do.
- Eat real food, mostly plants, and plenty of fish.
- Take vitamin D or cod liver oil. (Current formulations of cod liver oil no longer have too much Vitamin A and are therefore safe to use.)
- Take calcium supplements.
- Exercise regularly.
- Keep your WC in the safe range.
- Drink alcohol in moderation.
- Don't smoke.
- Don't do recreational drugs.
- Don't take unnecessary medications.

- Do take necessary or helpful medications exactly as prescribed.
- Avoid overexposure to the sun but get enough sunshine so that you make vitamin D.
- Be sure you have a large and close social network—the actual kind, not the virtual kind.
- Get enough sleep, including cat naps.
- Enjoy Smart Sex if you can.
- Analyze the sources of stress in your life and do everything you can to eliminate them.
- Have an annual physical.
- Get the preventive tests and shots you need in each decade of your life.
- Find time for pursuits that give you joy and a sense of fulfillment.
- Walk and climb stairs everywhere you can.
- Have goals and dreams no matter what your age.
- Help others.
- Have faith in a higher power. (Scientific studies have shown this will benefit your health!)
- Don't spend what you don't have or buy what you don't need.

Yet above all, live by my Golden Rule of Health for Women:

"Do unto yourself as you would do unto others."

Never neglect your own needs. As busy as you may be with your partner, your kids, your friends, your elderly parents, your pets, and your work, don't focus on those demands at the expense of your personal health. You're doing nobody any good if you put yourself at risk for diseases and conditions that you stand an excellent chance of avoiding simply by taking the Lifestyle Pill.

Do it for yourself. Do it for those you love. Do it for me.

—*Dr. Marie*

Index

Acknowledgments

My deepest appreciation goes to my late mother. She was a nurse who inspired me to follow in her footsteps. Her death after a long illness at the age of eighty-three came just as I was completing this book. May the many passages that I had already written about her guidance, wisdom, and encouragement stand as a testimony to a life well lived. Thanks, Mom.

While I was at the University of Pennsylvania, I had the support of my advisor, Dr. Helen Davies. She fought for me when I wanted to get into medical school because she believed that I was destined to be a doctor. During my training, Dr. John Eisenberg gave me the courage to look at issues from a global impact-outcomes perspective. Dr. Anne Marie Chirico, the first woman internist at Penn, showed me that it was possible for a woman doctor to be every bit as good if not better than a man. Dr. Sylvan Eisman taught me that patients are unique individuals who deserve to be treated as such.

I've always strived to do exactly that, and I want to thank all of my patients—the women, the men, the Cabrini nuns—who have taught me so much about the importance of caring instead of just curing.

Certainly, I also owe a debt of gratitude to my wonderful husband and my three terrific sons. Their respect for me and my work has always given me great hope that in the future we can raise a new generation of men, including male doctors, who will honor and value women whether as professionals, mothers, caregivers, or patients. Thank you Brad, Zach, Aaron, and Ben. You are simply the best family I could ever have.

Thanks also to my sister Eileen for being there with my parents as their health buddy. That has always given me great peace of mind. In addition, Eileen works tirelessly with me to get the word out about helping people take control of their own health care.

Acknowledgments

I'm grateful to ABC, where I am a Medical Contributor on *Good Morning America*, for giving me a larger stage from which to spread my message. Special thanks to ABC's Kerry Smith for her timely and astute review of the manuscript.

This book could not have come to fruition without the enthusiasm and expertise of my literary agent, Jane Dystel. She believed in me even through some rough stretches and gave me the confidence to write the book she knew I had in me.

I was fortunate indeed to have as my editor the very professional and equally personable Mary Norris at GPP Life. Her clear and judicious guidance has been invaluable from the first page to the last.

Finally my thanks go to my writing partner, Sondra Forsyth. We are joined at the hip when it comes to our shared passion for empowering patients with information. Sondra and I shared so much during the writing of our two previous books, and we brought all of that with us to this project. Right from the start, she immediately *got* my voice and my passion. She also added her own knowledge as a seasoned journalist specializing in women's issues including health, relationships, parenting, and sexuality. This book has truly been a collaboration—just like the one I wish for you in your partnership with your health-care providers as you strive to live long and well.

—Marie Savard, M.D.